John

27 – 11 – 1981

Springer Series on MEDICAL EDUCATION

Series Editor: Steven Jonas, M.D.
Series Advisers: Howard S. Barrows, M.D.
John Gordon Freymann, M.D.

A series designed to stimulate thought, discuss innovations, and present program evaluations in the field of medical education.

Howard S. Barrows, M.D., F.R.C.P.(C.), is a professor of medicine (neurology) and the director of Problem-Based Learning Systems, McMaster University, Faculty of Health Sciences.

Robyn M. Tamblyn, B. Sc.N., is a clinical lecturer in nursing and the associate director of Problem-Based Learning Systems, McMaster University, Faculty of Health Sciences.

Problem-Based Learning

An Approach to Medical Education

Howard S. Barrows, M.D.
Robyn M. Tamblyn, B.Sc.N.

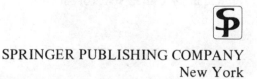

SPRINGER PUBLISHING COMPANY
New York

Springer Publishing Company, Inc.
200 Park Avenue South
New York, New York 10003

80 81 82 83 84 / 10 9 8 7 6 5 4 3 2 1

Library of Congress Cataloging in Publication Data

Barrows, Howard S.
    Problem-based learning.

    (Springer series on medical education ; 1)
    Bibliography: p.
    Includes index.
    1. Medicine, Clinical — Study and teaching. 2. Medical logic — Study and teaching. I. Tamblyn, Robyn M., joint author. II. Title. III. Series. [DNLM: 1. Education, Medical. 2. Learning. 3. Problem solving. W1 SP685SE v. 1 /W18 B278p]
R834.B37   616'.007'11   80-13429
ISBN 0-8261-2840-8
ISBN 0-8261-2841-6 (pbk.)

Printed in the United States of America

Contents

Foreword

With the publication of *Problem-Based Learning: An Approach to Medical Education* we are pleased to inaugurate the "Springer Series on Medical Education," a series of publications that will highlight new directions and point the way to change in this complex and vital area of human endeavor. The basic premise of "Medical Education" is indeed that change is needed in the medical education system. Thus books in the series will consider such subjects as curriculum planning and development; teaching methodology; the evaluation of teachers; the evaluation of students; the training of teachers; the politics, economics, and history of change in medical education; factors in medical student career planning; the teaching of new subjects in medical education; licensing, certification, quality assurance and medical education; and biomedical research policy and medical education.

Change is needed in medical education for several reasons. Although there are multiple loci of power in any health care delivery system, the physician is an important one. It is the physician who holds the medical license, who has a high degree of training in biomedical science, and who makes the decisions determining the majority of the expenditure of resources in the health care delivery system. Thus physicians control the keystones of the health care delivery system and have a very important influence on its character and mode of functioning. There are two major influences on the behavior of physicians: how they are trained and how they are paid. This series will deal with the former.

The problems of the health care delivery system are well known and need not be detailed here. Because of the centrality of the physician to the operations of the health care delivery system, it is obvious that the work of medical schools has an important relationship to the work of the system: it is the medical schools that both choose and train the physicians. The most important motivation to change in medical education, therefore, is that the problems of the health care delivery system must be attended to, and change in medical education can lead to solutions of at least some of those problems.

In *Problem-Based Learning,* Howard Barrows and Robyn Tamblyn address some basic problems in the learning of biomedical science, medicine, and the other health sciences. Students in most modern medical schools, especially in the basic science courses, are required to memorize a large number of "facts." Often the sets of facts they are required to memorize are chosen by the instructor based on what he or she knows and is familiar with. The sets of facts may or may not be relevant to medical practice. Furthermore, the student, a passive recipient in this approach, may or may not learn the facts in such a way that they are useful in future practice, regardless of whether the student is able to demonstrate on examination that his or her memory is good.

Problem-based learning has two fundamental postulates. The first is that learning through problem-solving is much more effective for creating in a student's mind a body of knowledge *usable* in the future than is traditional memory-based learning. The second is that the physician skills most important for patients are problem-solving skills, not memory skills. Most contemporary medical education provides students only limited opportunities to hone the general problem-solving skills with which their undergraduate education and life experiences have already equipped them. It consciously teaches little of the scientific method in biomedical problem-solving that is so much a part of good patient care. The problem-based learning approach, of course, has enormous utility for teaching in all the health sciences.

This book presents the scientific basis of problem-based learning in medical education. It then goes on to describe the approaches to problem-based medical learning that have been developed over the years at McMaster University. Barrows and Tamblyn are two of the principal creators of this "McMaster System." They have made a major contribution to the development of what will be the next historical stage of medical education. This book describes their work, in lucid and lively prose. We are proud to present it as the first in our "Springer Series on *Medical Education.*"

STEVEN JONAS, M. D.

Preface

In this book the term *problem-based learning* refers to a very specific approach to education in medicine, supported by tools designed to facilitate a specific teaching–learning process, all described in the subsequent chapters of this book. Problem-based learning is not simply the presentation of problems to students as a focus for learning or as an example of what has just been learned. As described in this book, it is a rigorous, structured approach to learning that is tailor-made for medical education and based on considerable experience and research.

The questions that need to be considered in this preface are: Why is problem-based learning necessary? What evidence is there for its effectiveness? The answers have come to me through the series of experiences that lead to this book being written.

In 1963, I had been responsible for several years for a neurological clinical clerkship through which six or more third-year medical students percolated every four weeks. I became concerned that the usual faculty evaluations were not providing data that were truly helpful to the student. As a result, the simulated patient was developed and used as a standardized patient problem; this provided more data concerning student competence (Barrows & Abrahamson, 1964). It revealed that, although students had, for the most part, good techniques in performing a neurological history and physical examination, they seemed to have a paucity of basic knowledge that they could apply to the patient problem. This seemed paradoxical to me, as I had been closely associated with, and contributed to, the students' prior courses in neuroanatomy, neurophysiology, and clinical neurology. I knew that these students had been exposed to, and had passed, excellent, detailed courses.

This observation about students was shared by many on the faculty, leading to the recurrent, half-serious suggestion that the school ought to have an "inverted curriculum" where the students would have two years of patient exposure and then two years of basic science. Students thus could enhance their learning and application of information, since the importance and relevance of basic science information could be perceived more readily.

George Miller (1962, 1978) has described on several occasions a study that documents the students' poor retention of basic science information. He asked sophomores, juniors, and seniors to retake the freshman examinations they had passed. It made no difference whether those students came from the upper or lower quarter of the class; none of them passed the retake. Miller has claimed that this retention of basic science information decreases at the same rate as has been shown for the retention of nonsense syllables. Levine and Forman (1973) went a step further and retested students about to enter their neurology clerkship. They were asked fifty questions that were chosen, because of their clinical relevance, from their first-year integrated neuroscience course. Almost two-thirds of the students received scores below minimum pass. Kelley West (1966) succinctly summarizes the fallacies of this traditional educational approach by pointing out that both logic and research prove it to be ineffective and, worse, inefficient.

Despite my realization that learning from patients and learning from books and teachers should go hand in hand, few substantial changes could be made in the curriculum of the school, despite endless efforts by a valiant but embattled group of faculty. As a result, I accepted the opportunity to take a sabbatical at McMaster University. My objectives were (1) to contribute to the efforts of a nuclear group that was designing a medical-school curriculum based solely on small-group, student-centered, individualized learning, and (2) to carry out personal study. During this sabbatical, my exposure to the teaching methods and concepts of Jim Anderson, a member of that nuclear group, provided me with considerable insight into the advantages of facilitatory teaching and the need to provide students with a packaged problem that would complement their work with simulated patients and real patients. This lead to the development, upon my return from sabbatical, of prototypes for neurology "problem boxes" for clinical clerks. Students found these units to be engrossing, motivating, a challenge to their clinical problem solving, and a useful stimulus for reviewing basic science information.

To determine the best design for the problem box and to evaluate and facilitate the students' clinical competence, it became necessary to obtain a better understanding of how practicing clinicians dealt with patient problems. The simulated patient as a standardized problem seemed an appropriate tool for such a study. In 1969, I had the opportunity to work briefly with Shulman and Elstein, who were also embarking on a study of the physician's medical inquiry skills and wanted to use simulated patients (Elstein et al., 1972; Elstein, Shulman, & Sprafka, 1978). Subsequently, with the help of Kara Bennett, I carried out a study of neurological residents, clinical clerks, and neurologists (Barrows & Bennett, 1972). We utilized the simulated patient and adapted Shulman and Elstein's technique of videotape recall (described in Chapter 2). I discovered that medical students and residents, for the most part, did not seem to think at all. Some gathered data ritualistically and then tried to add it up afterwards, while others came up with a diagnosis based on some symptom or sign, never considering possible alternatives. Subsequent experience with other students and other schools reinforced this uncomfortable observation and revealed even richer pathologies in thinking. Christine McGuire (1972) states that many medical schools would find that their graduates are wanting in clinical problem-solving skills, if they would use the appropriate tools to evaluate them. It seemed obvious to me at this point that students must learn, by working with problems, to develop appropriate problem-solving skills, and must make basic and clinical science learning more memorable and effective through their work with patients.

In 1971, I returned to McMaster and took advantage of what seemed to be an appropriate opportunity to develop the techniques of problem-based learning. My concepts appeared to fit well into their student-centered, small-group learning approach and seemed most relevant to their educational objectives (Neufeld & Barrows, 1974). A pilot program of totally problem-based learning was applied in the neuroscience portion of the curriculum, centered around some 22 problem boxes adapted from the neurology clerkship model. With the help of Donna Mitchell, my two-year experience with this approach was evaluated; its advantages seemed obvious (Barrows & Mitchell, 1975).

Evidence for the effectiveness of problem-based learning or "discovery" learning, has been in the literature for some time. Although the results of Katona (1940), Hilgard (1953), and Schmidt (1965), utilizing Katona's "card tricks," can be seen to be particularly relevant, they are not based on the use of patient problems. Moreover, any direct study of the advantages of problem-based learning in medicine requires comparison with a control group receiving more traditional educational experiences. This was not possible in the Barrows and Mitchell study. Tamblyn and I, however, had an unusual opportunity to attempt a study of the effects of problem-based, small-group learning on a small group of students within a more traditional curriculum and compare them with a similar control group. The experimental group demonstrated increased skills in problem formulation and self study, as well as a significantly greater motivation to seek clinical experience on their own (Barrows & Tamblyn, 1976a). On many subsequent occasions we have had the opportunity to engage student groups from many different schools in problem-based learning experience. Both the students and observing faculty are invariably impressed with the effects of this approach on both student motivation and learning.

In 1971, both Vic Neufeld and I felt that the inquiry studies of Shulman and Elstein's group and my study with Bennett could not provide generalizations about the problem-solving approach of the average physician and left many questions unanswered. With the assistance of Geoff Norman and John Feightner, we completed a study of 62 standardized patient encounters performed by a large number of general physicians selected at random. An analysis of extensive computerized data from this study allowed for a synthesis of the physician's problem-solving skills; this served as the model for the clinical problem-solving skills to be developed by medical students in problem-based learning (Barrows et al., 1978).

As a result, it was obvious to both Tamblyn and me that the problem boxes, as well as most other printed problem formats, were not challenging the student to develop all the important stages of the clinician's problem-solving approach. A specific problem was the linearity of these formats, which does not take into account the fact that the student should be free to take any action he wishes and in any sequence, as he can with actual patients, if he is to develop inquiry strategies. On a memorable day in October 1974, we watched a group of students become enthusiastically and totally involved in our first model of what has become known as the "P4," hastily written out by hand on various colored file cards. We were subsequently supported by a contract from the National Library of Medicine (No. 1-LM-6-4721) to produce and evaluate this format of problem-based learning units for neuroscience teaching. Rimoldi's (1973) prior work with a more limited version of a similar tool indicated that the student's problem-solving skills could be analyzed by this approach. Tamblyn's formal evaluation of this format with medical and nursing students suggested that this tool can be used by students, allows them to analyze and develop problem-solving skills, facilitates appropriate self-directed study, and, in addition, seems an attractive, motivating format (Tamblyn & Barrows, 1978).

Work with faculty and students from many schools in developing problem-based learning approaches has continued to demonstrate their effectiveness in helping students to develop scientific thinking about patients' problems and to acquire both basic science and clinical information in a manner that ensures retention and transfer to the real-life task of the clinician. Much more needs to be done to enhance the value of problem-based learning, to evaluate its strengths and weaknesses, and to give faculty and students skills in its employment. It is hoped that this book will make a contribution in this important area.

I would like to acknowledge my indebtedness to Steven Abrahamson and Jim Anderson for the education I have received working with them. The help I have received from Vic Neufeld, Geoff Norman, and the many others in the Program for Educational Development at McMaster must also be acknowledged. The continual support I have received working with Robyn

Tamblyn, carrying out many of the difficult but necessary aspects of work and study in problem-based learning, has allowed for a quantum jump in productivity. She has provided new insights into and techniques for problem-based learning. More importantly, she has worked to make this approach both relevant and available to other health professions, particularly nursing. In her own work, she has shown how effective problem-based learning can be for interdisciplinary education in health sciences; this is a most needed but, as yet, relatively unexplored area in health education. I also want to acknowledge the more-than-moral support I have received from my four daughters and from my wife, Phyllis. Not only have they tolerated my many trips around the countryside to work with teachers and students interested in problem-based learning and my eternal reading and writing at home, but they have provided constant encouragement and help. Lastly, both Robyn Tamblyn and I owe a great debt to Pearl Dodd, who has proofread, critiqued, and typed the manuscripts for this book countless times.

HOWARD S. BARROWS

For the purposes of clarity, this book has been written with a major focus on the experiences of problem-based learning in medical education. In reading this text, it is important to keep in mind that this teaching–learning format is both relevant and appropriate for the education of other health professionals (nursing, physiotherapy, occupational therapy, and so forth). The common factor among these disciplines is the need to actively apply knowledge to the assessment and care of patients and the ability to continue to identify areas where further learning would enhance or improve the practice of these skills. As in medicine, problem-based, student-centered learning is the most efficient method of simultaneously developing knowledge, reasoning skills, and study skills. Disciplines will differ in the problem situations they select for their students and the goals and expectations for patient assessment and care, but the basic learning method can be the same.

There are added benefits when the problem is used as the focus of study in team learning. The relationship between disciplines can be seen clearly and developed around an appropriate focus, the patient. Common and unique professional knowledge and skills can be observed and discussed and, in our experience, a more efficient and effective team relationship is a natural result.

ROBYN M. TAMBLYN

Introduction

Over the last few years, we have worked with faculty and students of many schools in North America, Holland, England, and Japan, in workshops devoted to problem-based learning, the use of simulated patients, and the design of problem-based learning units. This book has evolved from many requests for a basic text in the area. It represents both an update and an enlargement of a brief monograph we designed for faculty and students, to orient them to problem-based learning. It incorporates what we have learned from the experiences and studies described, as weil as the many ideas and comments we have gained from our various faculty and student interactions.

We have attempted to avoid jargon as much as possible. We offer no apologies for the fact that many of our educational researches and examples are in neurology; this is our field of expertise and our involvement in problem-based learning was due to attempts to accomplish more effective learning in neurology. It is our hope that the reader will see how the concepts and techniques described here can be useful in his or her teaching or learning, regardless of the subject matter. In an attempt to allow faculty and students in all varieties of teaching situations to see the relevance of this approach to their own needs, this text tries to avoid using one educational level, class size, or teacher-student relationship wherever possible. This may seem confusing to the reader unless it's appreciated that we want to concentrate on the *processes* involved in both student learning and the interaction between teacher and student, not on the particular student, teacher, or setting.

Although we have opted to use the male personal pronoun out of convenience, it is intended that she or he and her or his are completely interchangeable.

The structure of problem-based learning as a technique, the rationale for its use, the necessary tools, the teaching skills required, and techniques for evaluation will be described in considerable detail. It is our hope that the reader will find useful ideas in this book that can be expanded or adapted to meet his or her needs.

Definition of Terms

A brief definition of some terms seems in order here. Although most terms are defined in the context of the book, these few could seem mystifying or misinterpreted without comment at the outset on our specific use.

Teacher: This refers to anyone responsible for the education of students, for example, full-time faculty, part-time faculty, practicing physicians, other health professionals, or other students.

Students: This refers to anyone engaged in problem-based learning who wants to gain knowledge and skills, including medical students, interns, residents, physicians, nursing students, nurses, and so forth.

Clinician: This refers to anyone evaluating a patient problem, such as a physician, student, or nurse.

Diagnostic process: This refers to the analytical or evaluative process aimed at determining the cause or nature of a patient problem (as contrasted to therapeutic processes concerned with management or treatment). It does not refer to arriving at a specific or refined "diagnosis" or "differential diagnosis," which is often neither possible nor necessary.

Action: This term, for writing convenience, refers to any of a variety of actions, cognitive or physical, made by the clinician in his evaluation and treatment of the patient. Actions include asking questions of the patient, examining the patient, ordering laboratory or diagnostic tests, requesting consultation, treating the patient, talking to relatives, asking for patient records, and the like.

CHAPTER 1

Problem-Based Learning: Rationale and Definition

Learning from problems is a condition of human existence. In our attempts to solve the many problems we face every day, learning occurs. In looking for offices in an unfamiliar building, or addresses in an unfamiliar town, we eventually find our way. In filling out income tax statements, learning occurs, just as in trying to find out why the car won't start. Although we may not be consciously aware, these problem situations are all learning experiences that are providing us with information and knowledge that we can apply to future problems. The more opportunity we have to use this information in our day-to-day activities, the more ingrained and unforgettable it becomes. We may recall occasions when we have provided a friend or colleague with very helpful and even sophisticated information about a problem he is attempting to solve. Although that information may seem to have just "popped" into our mind as our friend attempted to solve his problem, a little reflection will reveal that we acquired it from our own experience with a similar problem. No doubt, problem-based learning is the basic human learning process that allowed primitive man to survive in his environment. Facts related to us by others or information we have read ourselves rarely seem to have the tenacity of the information we have gained from our own daily confrontation with problems. It would be safe to say that the great wealth of information we possess in our memory banks has remained there as a consequence of having worked with problems we have been faced with in such life situations as school, work, social situations, and our hobbies. Problem-based learning is the learning that results from the process of working toward the under-standing or resolution of a problem. The problem is encountered *first* in the learning process!

There is nothing new about the use of problem solving as a method of learning in a variety of educational settings. Unlike what occurs in real-life situations, however, the problem usually is not given to the student first, as a stimulus for active learning. It usually is given to the student after he has been provided with facts or principles, either as an example of the importance of this knowledge or as an exercise in which the student can apply this knowledge.

Education as a Teaching Skill

Medical teachers will agree that medicine is a profession that requires, as a principle skill or capability, the lifelong ability to work through difficult and often unique patient problems. Despite this, the potential value or relevance of problem-based learning is not considered by teachers in their headlong rush to expose students, during their brief years of formal medical education, to more and more of the ever-enlarging and complex body of important concepts and facts in the basic and clinical sciences. In fact, the careful design and development of better educational methods, or approaches to medical education, is usually given a low priority by those involved in medical education. The reasons for all of this may be easy to understand.

Characteristically, teachers responsible for both the design of medical educational programs and for teaching the students in these programs, have other, more demanding responsibilities, usually in the areas of research and clinical service. Each member of a medical faculty has spent many arduous years gaining the knowledge and skills necessary to successfully carry out tasks in research and patient care. Few have taken the time to gain any specific or formal preparation to aid them in carrying out their responsibilities in medical education. While this is considered acceptable, medical schools would not tolerate such an amateur status in those responsible for research or patient care.

Without a background of specific studies or experiences in the applied sciences of education, medical faculty must draw upon their past experiences as students as a model for their own concepts and behaviors regarding education. This is shortsighted, however, since these faculty are responsible for the education of large numbers of students who will become the future providers of medical care and research. In the long view, as faculty, teaching should be their greatest responsibility. The fact that they are faculty in a medical *school* should indicate that education is a primary task. The reasons for this paradoxical situation are a matter of history and reflect the reward system used in medical schools, where faculty development in education is not encouraged. There are few schools who would put the education of students as their highest priority, or who would allow faculty promotion and remuneration to reflect educational knowledge and skills equal to or above research and patient-care productivity. Nevertheless, if medical faculty would apply to the education of students the same skills of inquiry, reasoning, and treatment design they use in patient care and research, their amateur status in education would soon disappear and students would profit.

This perspective provides the rationale for this book, which was designed as a guide to medical education as an applied science, for those medical teachers who are interested in investigating better ways to prepare their students for the tasks they will have to perform as physicians. It is also intended that the approaches described here will be useful to other health science disciplines. To this end, the authors have drawn upon their additional experiences with nursing, physiotherapy, and social work students, as well as faculty in both unidisciplinary and multidisciplinary learning situations. The thesis of this book is that problem-based learning represents the appropriate educational method for medical students if their educational needs are considered from a logical or scientific point of view.

The Objectives of Medical Education

A basic concern for any educational program is whether or not the teaching or learning methods presently in use are appropriate to the outcomes expected of students. This is the same question that has to be answered in selecting a treatment plan for a patient or in choosing an experimental research method. There is a wide variety of teaching–learning options; the choice depends on the desired outcomes, which are the objectives of medical education.

Since the medical student is to become a physician, the expected outcomes can be identified by defining the tasks a physician is expected to perform competently. In the authors' opinion, the principle requirement of any physician, implied by the M.D. degree, can be stated as follows: *The physician should be able to evaluate and manage patients with medical problems effectively, efficiently, and humanely.*

Some of the terms used in this statement need to be elaborated so that the range of competencies assumed can be appreciated better.

Evaluate: This term encompasses a variety of subskills, such as the cognitive skills of clinical reasoning or medical problem solving, as well as interview, physical examination, and interpersonal skills.

Manage: This term implies skills in the selection and application of appropriate therapeutic interventions, such as medication, surgery, counseling, rehabilitation, and patient education in acute and chronic conditions. Clinical problem-solving or reasoning skills also are involved in this activity.

Patient: This term refers to anyone who either directly requests the physician's services or is referred to the physician for an identified or suspected health problem.

Medical: This term refers to the specific component of health care that belongs to the physician. It recognizes that the physician is a member of a team with many specialists, including nurses, rehabilitation therapists, psychologists, nutritionists, social workers, and so forth. Psychiatry is considered a medical discipline in this definition.

Effectively: This term refers to the accuracy and appropriateness of the physician's evaluation and care of the patient. The patient evaluation should be as precise and adequate as the time, urgency, and data available from the patient allow. The management of the problem should be appropriate to the particular patient and his particular problem.

Efficiently: This term implies an appropriate use of time and costs. The physician should not spend an hour with a problem that should only require fifteen minutes, nor should he use hundreds of dollars on laboratory tests and investigations when a less expensive workup would suffice. This definition also refers to his use of medical facilities and other health professionals.

Humanely: This term requires that the physician should be concerned about the patient as a person and not as a medical problem or disease. His evaluation and management should reflect an awareness of the patient's cultural, familial, economic, and psychological needs.

This task statement for the physician can be adapted and modified to be appropriate for such particular sectors of medical practice such as primary care, secondary care, general or family practice, or specialty practice. It serves, however, as a useful orientation to the behavior we would like to see medical students demonstrate upon graduation.

The next important task for the physician relates to his medical career. No matter where the physician finds himself working in medicine, which is a vast, dynamic profession with many specialties, subdisciplines and a variety of practice settings, his own particular area of practice or specialty will be subjected constantly to new information, new concepts, new techniques and new problems. The hundreds of specialty journals that arrive each month at the medical libraries and the increasing size of each year's medical indices are mute testimony to this fact. The important new knowledge that each physician will need to know in the future is unknown now. Some of the facts he has learned as a student in his formal years of medical education will no longer be useful to him in the future because they will be obsolete or incorrect. Neither faculty nor students will ever be able to predict which facts these will be (West, 1966). Only a portion of what is taught in medical school will be relevant to the particular career in medicine that the student enters as a physician. As a consequence, the physician must continue to learn the rest of his life if he is to be effective, safe, and relevant. Almost all of the learning a physician will need to accomplish in his forty or more years of professional work, after his formal medical education, will be his own responsibility.

The logical second task for the physician, therefore, is to continuously evaluate his own abilities, determine when new skills and knowledge are needed, and effectively use available resources to meet these identified needs. This can be stated as follows: *The physician should be able to continuously define and satisfy his particular educational needs in order to keep his skills and information contemporary with his chosen field and to care properly for the medical problems he encounters.*

If this latter task had been made a priority at medical schools decades ago, the contemporary problems of continuing medical education, recertification, and peer reviews might not be of such magnitude now. Instead, the objective of many medical schools, intended or not, is to ensure that the students become walking encyclopedias of medical knowledge in order to achieve high marks on certifying examinations. We hope that this will shift soon to an emphasis on gaining secure skills in patient evaluation, patient management, and self study.

Vocational versus Scholarly Knowledge

It is unfortunate that many medical school teachers consider the tasks we have just discussed, especially the evaluation and management of the patient's medical problem, to be vocational skills. Their feeling is that these skills would be more appropriately addressed in clinical clerkships, clinical electives, and postgraduate or residency education, and that the responsibility of the undergraduate educational program should be to ensure that the student acquires a firm knowledge base in the basic and clinical sciences. In their opinion, therefore, a physician should be a scholar in the medical sciences and the mission for a medical school is to produce such scholars.

This justifiable concern for a sound knowledge base in the basic sciences and medical specialties has led to a preoccupation with the delivery of content and with measurements of its retention by recall on such objective examinations as the national boards. Scores on these examinations have become the criteria for student and even medical school excellence. As important and essential as this knowledge is, however, its relationship to the purposes of a medical education is distorted. It is important for teachers to realize that the evaluation and management of health problems, whether you call it medical problem solving or the clinical reasoning process, is the physician's *science* (see Chapter 2 for more detail). This science is definable, amenable to evaluation, and has the potential for being improved upon by appropriate teaching. Basic and clinical science knowledge in medicine must be developed in relationship to the acquisition of this skill.

A student's acquisition of a large body of knowledge in medicine and the basic sciences is no assurance that he knows when or how to apply this knowledge in the care of patients. There is little evidence that the amount of factual knowledge possessed by a student, as scored by objective examinations, correlates in any way with clinical competence (Wingard & Williamson, 1973). A consistently competent clinical performance by a student does ensure, however, that he possesses adequate factual knowledge. This was concisely stated by George Miller, who wrote, "the best performance is built upon sound information; but the provision, or even the acquisition, of sound information is no assurance that it will occur" (Miller, 1967a). In order to solve a problem in mathematics or physics, facts and principles have to be learned. Similarly, great amounts of information have to be acquired in the basic sciences and clinical medicine in order for a physician to evaluate and manage medical problems (Pauker et al., 1976). No scholarship in medical science should be sacrificed through concern for the student's acquisition of clinical problem-solving skills, but it is important that the information is acquired in a manner that permits application to the problems faced by the physician.

Perhaps the appropriate relationship of content knowledge to professional skill or process in medical education might be seen more clearly if an analogy were made to another profession. Commercial aviation is a profession that, like medicine, requires complex skills and public accountability for the pilot's competency. Imagine that you are about to enter a commercial aircraft and that you are told that the pilot has just graduated from a commercial aviation school. To reassure you about this new graduate's competence in the field of aviation, you are told of the important sciences basic to aviation that he has been taught, including physics of flight, geophysics, aircraft design, meteorology, navigation, aircraft engine design and function, hazards in flight, airport design, and so on. To further reassure you of his ability to fly this aircraft you are told that he was given a whole battery of multiple-choice questions and that he had received high marks. He was even given problems on paper, to determine what he would do if an engine failed or a wing was damaged; he handled them very well. It seems doubtful that you would be reassured, despite his scholarship in aviation science, unless you were told that he had proved his proficiency in actual flight maneuvers. Your real concern would relate to his ability to take off, his competency to fly, his ability to get you safely to your destination, and to land. You would hope he could competently handle any unsuspected, real-life problems or emergencies that might develop during your flight.

If we look in the same manner at medicine, a profession with high public accountability, it seems to us that there should be little argument that

1. The physician should be able to evaluate and manage patients with medical problems effectively, efficiently, and humanely (clinical reasoning).
2. The physician should be able to continually define and satisfy his particular educational needs in order to keep his skills and information contemporary with his chosen field and to care properly for the problems he encounters (self-evaluation and study).

The emphasis in medical education, therefore, must be on the *application* of knowledge.

Competencies

Selecting Appropriate Teaching–Learning Options

There are many other tasks that the physician must perform in his professional activities, whether they be at the bedside, in the clinic, in the hospital, among his peers, with other health professionals, or in the community. Medical faculties must identify all the tasks they want their graduates to acquire and identify them as objectives of medical education. The relative priority and weight of each task determines the criteria by which the most appropriate teaching–learning techniques can be selected and implemented.

The possible teaching–learning methods in medicine can be conveniently categorized in two ways. The first categorization is based on the person responsible for making the decisions of what the student is to learn. Is it the teacher (teacher-centered) or the student (student-centered)? The second category is based on how the body of knowledge and skills is organized for learning. Does it center on subject areas (subject-based) or problem areas (problem-based)? A curriculum can be teacher-centered/subject-based, student-centered/subject-based, teacher-centered/problem-based or student-centered/problem-based.

Teacher-Centered Learning

In this method, the teacher is solely responsible for what the student is expected to learn. The teacher decides what information and skills the student should learn, how it is to be learned, in what sequence, and at what pace. It is a well-known model that we have been exposed to since kindergarten. Although the teacher's usual role in this method is to dispense information in lectures, assign readings and provide demonstrations, a modular, self-study or individualized learning curriculum also can be teacher-centered if the teacher determines the modules or resources that are to be studied, the sequence of study, and the learning that is to be mastered. The characteristic that identifies a teacher-centered curriculum is that the student is not responsible for his own education.

Advantages.   Experts in specialty or basic science disciplines often find themselves with heavy research and patient-care responsibilities and little time for teaching. In these instances, a teacher-centered curriculum is an ideal format. The expert can readily dispense to the students information and insights gained through his own work in his field through the use of lectures, seminars, monographs, and reading assignments. The teacher can be certain that the student is exposed to all the knowledge and concepts he feels are appropriate for learning. It is easy for a person who has worked many years in a field to synthesize difficult subjects into easily digested capsules, making this a most efficient method for dispensing content knowledge. It saves the student the agony, frustration, and time that would be squandered if he were forced to work through the subject areas on his own.

This is the educational method universally recognized by students, teachers, and administrators. Success as a teacher in this format depends on one's knowledge as an expert and one's flair for dispensing this knowledge. This flair can be expressed in the organization, the insights provided and humor incorporated in the lectures, and in the learning resources used.

Disadvantages.   Students are not homogeneous in background, knowledge, or experience, nor are they homogeneous in their learning abilities in different areas or in their pace and style of learning. Each has different career aspirations. In teacher-centered learning, the teacher imposes what he assumes all students should know, without regard to variations in ability, need, or comprehension of new data.

The student is a passive recipient in this method and does not learn to dig it out for himself or "learn to learn." His task is to learn what is offered and to regurgitate it on demand. The students' rewards in teacher-centered learning are usually external, as motivation is invariably based on grades and not on personal desire for accomplishment (Knowles, 1975). Since examinations in this format are centered around the teacher's concept of what is to be learned, the evaluation process is also based on the teacher and not the student. As a consequence, the student does not learn how to evaluate himself against his own concept of what he feels should be learned.

This system makes heavy demands on the teacher, as he must constantly update and revise his material for lectures, readings, or syllabi so that the information he offers to his students is current.

Students and teachers can obtain a false sense of security if they believe that, once information is dispensed and a cognitive framework provided, the student will incorporate the information, recognize where and when it could and should be used, and apply it effectively at that time. Teacher-based learning may be seen as the most efficient method to cover the content to be learned, but it is the most inefficient method to meet the goals in self-evaluation and self-study. In addition, the student is seldom given the opportunity to apply the content learned until after he has graduated, when supervision and assistance are not always readily available.

The final disadvantage in teacher-based learning is that no one can predict which parts of the information the student has learned will eventually become obsolete or incorrect, what the student will forget, or what new information he will need to know in the future (West, 1966). We all can enumerate many important new concepts, skills, techniques, and diseases that have surfaced since we graduated from school.

Student-Centered Learning

In this method, the student learns to determine what he needs to know. Although the teacher may have considerable responsibility in the beginning, by providing the student with the necessary experience and guidance, it is expected that the student will eventually take full responsibility for his own learning. The emphasis is on active acquisition of information and skills by the student, depending on his ability to identify his educational needs, his best manner of learning, his pace of learning, and his ability to evaluate his learning. The teacher is available for guidance as needed until the student gains full independence.

In both the student-centered and the teacher-centered methods, the teacher may prepare what he feels are the appropriate learning objectives, learning resources, and evaluation materials that reflect his particular experience and knowledge. In the teacher-centered approach these materials prescribe exactly what the student is to learn. In the student-centered approach these materials serve as guides and resources to be used and adapted as the student feels appropriate, for taking on the responsibility for his education.

Advantages. In this method, the student does "learn to learn," so that he can meet a lifetime need to adapt to the new knowledge, challenges, and problems he will encounter in the future. He can make his present learning relevant to his educational needs, his future career, and his style and manner of learning, and can pace his learning appropriately, according to his ability to learn or understand in any particular area.

Since his learning is self-determined and acquired through his own "digging" or study, the student becomes an active participant in the learning process. This provides motivation. More important, what he learns is better retained, because he alone determines what is important to his own study, and seeks out the information himself. His rewards are internal: the desire to learn for personal or professional growth, not for teacher-dispensed rewards.

As the student is responsible for his own education, he also is responsible for the evaluation of his educational goals. The student acquires the ability to evaluate his own strengths and weaknesses, to determine his needs and to learn to meet these needs. The student, with guidance, has to establish his own criteria and methods of evaluation.

The educational work in this format is done by the student. He has the burden of finding up-to-date references or learning resources to meet his needs, using books, monographs, audiovisual resources, and faculty. As a physician, he will have to do this all his life, so it is important that he learn the skill now, during his formal education. The teacher plays a critical, facilitating role, but his main task is to eventually make himself redundant or dispensable to the student's progress. The student learns from the library, laboratory, faculty, and audiovisual resources, thus eliminating the need for endless syllabi, manuals, and reference lists to be prepared by teachers.

Disadvantages.   Student-based learning presents a number of organizational problems. Extensive learning resources must be available to the student (books, reprints, slides, videotapes, films, models, specimens, microscopes, cadavers, and so on) so that he can easily pursue his own individual needs. Problems occur because the curriculum must be unstructured in order to allow the student to spend time using the available resources, as he feels appropriate, in order to meet his own educational designs.

Evaluation has to be individualized. The convenience of providing one test for the whole class has to be abandoned. Each student must be evaluated against his own goals. The whole approach to evaluation has to change so that the student is allowed to set his own criteria for success. This is an educational advantage to the student, but the freedom allowed may be seen as a disadvantage to the teacher. There are, of course, certain non-negotiable goals that a medical school must require of its students, if that school is to fulfill its responsibility to the public. The student, by accepting a position in the school, must expect that there will be a number of competencies he will have to possess upon graduation.

This approach can create insecurity on the part of both students and faculty. In the beginning, the student worries about his ability to determine what he needs to know and to what depth. Many faculty cannot imagine how the student can learn on his own and are concerned that he may not learn all that is felt to be important. The student-centered approach requires maturity and discipline on the part of the student and a different order of educational skills for the teacher, who must be able to facilitate, guide, and evaluate the student as an individual learner, responsible for his own education. These are, however, qualities that the student, in his eventual role as a physician, must possess. What better time to develop them than medical school, where their effective growth can be monitored and enhanced by teachers?

Subject-Based Learning

In this most familiar method, the learning is organized around a subject area or field of learning in medicine or the basic sciences, such as anatomy, pharmacology, biochemistry, laboratory medicine, surgery, pediatrics, or neurology. Learning may be organized into a hierarchy of basic concepts that build up to more advanced concepts. The objective is for the student to gain an overall grasp of the subject area involved, to learn its important concepts in sufficient depth, to have an understanding of the field itself, or to apply concepts from that field to his future task as a physician. Again, this method is independent of the format, since subject-based learning can be individualized and self-paced. It does lend itself well to larger classroom approaches. It can be either student- or teacher-centered, as long as learning is organized around a subject.

Advantages. In this system, the end points or limits to student learning are defined by the subject area, as is the sequence of learning. The extent and depth of knowledge to be acquired is more easily defined for the students and the teacher.

Resources for learning in one specified subject or field are more easily identified and made available for student use. Teachers have more confidence in specifying all concepts and skills they feel need to be learned by the students.

This approach seems efficient, since the student applies himself to the task of memorizing and/or manipulating the concepts, skills, and information that are important, quickly and directly. Evaluation is easily designed to sample the student's recall of the specified knowledge and concepts identified, through the use of convenient and well-established tests (multiple-choice, true-false, word fill-in, and essay examinations). The student's successful recall of information provides both the teacher and the student with a feeling of security that adequate learning has occurred. This can be a disadvantage in that the student may feel immunized against any need for further learning in the subject area.

Disadvantages. The information learned in this approach can be reinforced only by experiences that require recall of the information learned. In subject-based learning this information is not readily recalled or reinforced by work with patients, since it is learned in association with an organized subject. Generations of students in conventional curricula have expressed the desire to repeat basic science courses when they enter their clinical years, testimony to their frustration over the inability to recall subject-based information from earlier years.

In subject-based learning, the information acquired is not conveniently integrated with information from other disciplines or subject areas. Even in so-called "integrated curricula," the student is exposed to juxtaposed information with no central focus around which to organize in his memory, except for the subject or course.

Although this method enhances the memorization and understanding of a large body of information in one subject area, it does not ensure that the student will be able to select in a problem situation the item of information from the specific discipline that will be helpful to him. The types of problems he will encounter as a physician will require the integration of many bits of information and skills from a variety of disciplines. If the cognitive connections among subjects are not actively laid down during the learning process, one cannot expect the student to intuitively develop these connections when faced with a patient problem where information from a variety of disciplines has potential application. How can subject-based learning be considered efficient in the long run if patients do not present themselves as isolated examples of information from one discipline?

This method of learning tends to reward the good memorizer and often inhibits the student who likes to learn by reasoning or inquiry. This latter skill often is not stressed in subject-based learning, yet it is a necessary cognitive behavior for the practicing physician.

Problem-Based Learning

In this approach, the student takes on a patient problem, a health delivery problem, or a research problem as a stimulus for learning in the areas, subjects, or disciplines that are appropriate for the student at the time. In doing this, the student exercises or further develops his problem-solving skills. This method of learning has two educational objectives: the acquisition of an integrated body of knowledge related to the problem, and the development or application of problem-solving skills.

Problem-based learning is ideally suited for student-centered and individualized learning. It can be used, however, in teacher-centered learning. The teacher can specify the problem to be used, the areas of study, and the resources or subjects to be studied relevant to the problem. This will develop students' problem-solving skills and involve them in the active acquisition of knowledge, but they are not challenged to learn for themselves. The term problem-based learning, as used here, implies student-centered learning as well.

Advantages. This approach is tailor-made for medicine. It provides advantages for both the acquisition of knowledge and the development of essential skills in patient problem solving. Information, concepts, and skills learned by the student are put into his memory in association with a problem. This allows the information to be recalled more easily when he faces another problem in which the information is relevant. Recall is constantly reinforced and elaborated by subsequent work with other problems. The student is able to use the problem as a focus for the study of many different subjects, actively integrating this information into a system that can be applied to the problem at hand and to subsequent problems.

By working with an unknown problem, the student is forced to develop problem-solving, diagnostic, or clinical reasoning skills. He must get information, look for cues, analyze and synthesize the data available, develop hypotheses, and apply strong deductive reasoning to the problem at hand. This approach is very motivating to students; medical students especially like to work with and solve patient problems, since this challenges them with the very situations they will face in their elected professional field.

Many studies have suggested that the effectiveness of the physician's diagnostic or clinical reasoning skills correlates directly with the experience and learning gained from prior patient problems. This is another endorsement for problem-based learning, since learning with this format requires the students' active participation in a large number of health problems.

When his learning is centered around patient problems, the student can see the relevance of what he has to learn, particularly the importance of basic science information to his future tasks. Problem-based learning will teach a skill that will continue to be useful to the student's professional life, where patients become the stimulus for further learning.

An added reward to problem-based/student-centered learning is the inevitable discovery, by teachers who become comfortable with this approach, that this method is enjoyable, rewarding, more natural, and actually takes less time. In student-centered work, the student carries out much of what was teacher activity. This approach is further enhanced by the responses seen in students. They become excited, motivated, evidence more mature behavior (they are being treated as self-determining adults), evolve secure clinical reasoning and learning skills, and acquire an impressive groundwork of basic knowledge.

Disadvantages. The success of problem-based/student-centered learning depends on students disciplining themselves to work with an unknown and possibly puzzling problem in a way that will challenge the development of their problem-solving skills and stimulate relevant self-directed learning. The teacher must have the skills necessary to orient and guide students in this process and to design as well as produce or assemble problem-based learning materials (see Chapter 9).

There are several concerns that often weaken the perceived value of problem-based learning. The first is the feeling that this method stresses the clinical concepts of patient evaluation and management, to the detriment of learning in the basic sciences. The second is that this method seems to stress problem-solving skills and not the acquisition of knowledge or facts. Both are unfounded if problem-based learning is correctly implemented. Experience has shown that students, if properly oriented and guided by medical teachers, can learn basic or clinical science in any area and to any depth. The challenge in working with a patient problem does not have to be the diagnosis or differential diagnosis of the problem. It just as easily can be to identify the underlying anatomical, biochemical, or physiological mechanisms involved in the problem and to understand how they function. The most important factor in the student's effective use of the problem is a clear understanding of the educational objectives of the program or unit. This provides both students and teachers with guidelines as to what possible areas they should pursue in working with the problems they have decided to use.

A third concern is that problem-based learning seems to be an inefficient way to learn. When confronted with an unfamiliar problem, the student requires considerable time to understand the terminology; the significance of symptoms or signs; the basic anatomy and physiology of the organ systems involved; and the social, epidemiological, or psychological dynamics in the problem. There are so many important and relevant areas that could be studied in any problem, it may seem as though an inordinate amount of time must be spent to complete the first problem in a new area. In actual fact, there is little inefficiency, since much of this study provides the factual groundwork for understanding other problems. As the student begins to grasp the basics, he moves more swiftly with subsequent problems on the knowledge he has gained from the first, while constantly reinforcing what has been learned.

This method of learning does not facilitate the student's ability to pass certifying examinations (national boards, multiple-choice, true-false) that largely stress recall of isolated facts and concepts. Recall occurs best for the student in this system when he is faced with a problem, not when he is faced with subject-oriented questions. Problem-based learning requires different types of examination tools that evaluate the student's ability to work with problems and apply learned information to their understanding or resolution (see Chapter 7). Many of the techniques and measurement tools used are unfamiliar and may seem "soft" to many teachers.

For both the teacher and the student, this approach requires considerable attention to learning objectives, identification of appropriate educational issues, and knowledge of the physician's cognitive processes and how they should be learned and evaluated.

Summary

It could be assumed easily that teacher-based learning refers to lectures and that student-based learning refers to individualized or self-directed study. There is no doubt that teacher-based learning is easiest with the lecture format and student-based learning can be facilitated best by self-study units of one type or another. It is important, however, to see these approaches as independent of format. The lecture can be student-based if students ask you to give a lecture on a subject they have decided is important for their learning at a particular point. Self-study units can be teacher-based if the teacher determines the units to be studied by the students, specifies the reading and other experiences that should be undertaken, the time to be taken, and gives an examination at the end to see if the students have learned what was felt by the teacher to be important.

The Appropriate Teaching/Learning Combination for Medicine

Certainly the most common combination of teaching and learning that occurs in medical schools is teacher-centered and subject-based. Knowles (1975) points out that teacher-centered, subject-based learning assumes that the learner's experience in learning is of less value than the teacher's. He also points out that the real competencies needed by students in teacher-centered, subject-based learning are to listen attentively, take careful notes, read rapidly with comprehension, predict examination questions, and be able to cram. He states that all that is required of the student in this method "is that he learns the material presented to him, and that he is able to reproduce it as accurately as possible on demand. As long as the product, i.e. precise re-production, is correct, we are satisfied." West (1966) adds, "In general the atmosphere of a great many if not most, American medical schools appears to be one in which the faculty assumes responsibility for presenting a common body of subject matter to all students and the students assume the responsi-bility for repeating it on demand."

If the educational program is built around lectures, it is important to recognize that they cannot be delivered at the convenience of the learner, nor can they be given at a level, pace, and priority important for the individual learner in the class. Lectures are often unrelated to any active application by the student and, by the time he needs the information given, it is forgotten. In fact, George Miller (1962) points out that, before they graduate, medical students forget most of what they learn in traditionally taught first-year anatomy and biochemistry. Knowledge *used* is better remembered.

When problem-based/student-centered learning is considered, however, the teacher's concern is that the method seems inefficient. This displays a blindness to a crucial issue: It is more important to consider how much the student learns than how much the teacher teaches. Typically, teacher-centered learning is concerned with transmission of content by the teacher. Student-centered learning is concerned with the acquisition of content by the student. In problem-based/student-centered learning, not only is knowledge acquired but skills in *using* knowledge are acquired (Knowles, 1975).

Perhaps one of the most important advantages of student-centered learning is that the student is motivated by the internal rewards of learning and not by the artifical or external rewards of grades. This produces a different climate in a medical school. The students are "turned on" constantly, they assist each other, and an informal collaborative relationship with faculty ensues. In addition, their learning is motivated by personal satisfaction, which will always be present, even when grades and passing exams are no longer an issue.

If we expect a student to develop (1) the ability to evaluate and manage patients with medical problems effectively, efficiently, and humanely (clinical reasoning skills) and (2) the ability to define and satisfy his particular educational needs to keep his skills contemporary with his chosen field and to care properly for the problems he encounters (self-directed study skills), it seems obvious that problem-based/student-centered education should be the principal method employed in medical school. Alternative techniques simply cannot compete with this method when it is realized that problem-based learning is the one that will help the student develop medical problem-solving skills. Additionally, it is the only method that ensures that the content learned is related to the task of resolving problems, reinforced in the student's memory by reuse with multiple patient problems, and made useful to the problem solver by the active and ongoing integration of information from many disciplines. The generalization of the principles learned with each problem ensures transfer of information and skills to the student's work with subsequent problems. Only student-centered learning will help the student to "learn to learn," a lifetime need for his professional work.

Faculty Members as Problem-Based Learners

Although there is a growing body of literature documenting the value of problem-based learning in education, we as teachers only need to reflect here on how we continue to learn and acquire information. All of us attempt to stay abreast of the literature in our particular area of specialty or expertise. We voraciously read our monthly journals and attend conferences and seminars, yet, most of the material covered in these endeavors is soon forgotten. If we run into a complex or difficult patient case or research problem, however, and have to read, talk to experts for advice, or research the literature for help, the information we gain invariably is far better retained. When you face another problem that is similar, it all floods back into your awareness, sometimes it seems as if by magic. In the study of the physician's problem-solving skills that will be described in the next chapter, it was not an infrequent occurrence for a physician suddenly to recall from his memory a sophisticated package of information to help evaluate or manage the patient problem he encountered. If you ask how he did it, he invariably will recall a case, a patient, or a similar problem he worked with months or years ago. Whenever a bright idea suddenly occurs to you in your work, reflect; it probably came from a previous problem. The journal, convention, and seminar approaches are teacher-centered and often subject-based. The puzzling over a problem in work is obviously problem-based/student-centered, self-directed learning. If it works so well for us, why not share it with our students?

However, experienced professionals probably learn more useful information from subject-based approaches, such as lectures and journals, than do students. They have a backlog of patient experiences and problems that can make the information relevant and its application in future use easily perceived.

Problem-Based Learning for Team Learning

Problem-based learning provides a potent format for interprofessional learning in the health sciences. Since the patient and his problem are the focus for health-care delivery, around which all members of the team perform, a problem can serve as an organizing structure for students from various professions to develop an understanding of each others' concerns and skills and to develop a team approach. They can discuss the concept each has of the patient's problem and how these fit together. They each can use the problem as motivation for study of the relevant areas from their own professional discipline and then decide on management and the appropriate use of their individual or complementary roles. We have had very productive experiences with problem-based learning for medical-student/nursing-student learning and for nurse/physiotherapist/physician team learning.

This emphasis on the advantage of problem-based learning does not mean that it is the only method appropriate in medical education, but that it should be a principal or major method. There are many occasions where other methods may meet certain educational objectives better; however, the usual employment of teacher-centered/subject-based learning as the principal or major method is not appropriate.

The Challenge of Applying Problem-Based Learning

With the rationale for problem-based learning in medical education now fully discussed, the focus of this book becomes the practical application of this technique. Teacher-centered/subject-based approaches are completely familiar to all of us, and we would have little difficulty in designing, selecting, or carrying out the educational activities needed in this approach, such as objectives, teaching methods, learning resources, and evaluation methods. Problem-based learning and self-directed learning, however, offer a new set of challenges in selecting, designing, and carrying out these functions. Facilitatory teaching skills are required. Problem-based learning units that are separate from learning resources are needed. Simulations of patient problems are needed to maximize the problem-based learning experience. Different evaluation tools to analyze the student's process of problem solving or clinical reasoning are required. A restructuring of time and teacher use may be needed. The task of this book will be to provide a more detailed discussion of these areas. In doing this, we hope to show how education can be an applied science where one uses the same logic as applied to research and patient care.

In summary, problem-based learning can be defined best as the learning that results from the process of working toward the understanding or resolution of a problem. The problem is encountered first in the learning process and serves as a focus or stimulus for the application of problem-solving or reasoning skills, as well as for the search for or study of information or knowledge needed to understand the mechanisms responsible for the problem and how it might be resolved. The problem is not offered as an example of the relevance of prior learning or as an exercise for applying information already learned in a subject-based approach. A problem in this context refers to an unsettled, puzzling, unsolved issue that needs to be resolved. It is a situation that is unacceptable and needs to be corrected. Finding the answer to a question is not problem-based learning. The use of a known principle or solution to explain an observation or phenomenon is not problem-based learning. The most frequently used problems are patient problems, which need not be classical diagnostic entities or even resolved problems in order to be useful. Problems other than patient problems also can be used to stimulate student reasoning and learning. Evaluation of research results or journal articles, health-care-delivery problems, medical research problems, hospital or practice administrative problems, team function problems, and so forth, all can be used to achieve appropriate objectives in medical education.

CHAPTER 2

The Clinical Reasoning Process: Problem Solving in Medicine

Background

The most important set of abilities the physician must possess are those involved in the clinical reasoning process. This term refers to the cognitive process that is necessary to evaluate and manage a patient's medical problems. This process is quite similar, if not identical, to the hypothetico-deductive reasoning process attributed to scientists working within their particular disciplines. The clinical reasoning process should be considered the "scientific method" of clinical medicine. Although many terms have been used to describe this cognitive process, such as medical problem solving, medical inquiry, clinical judgment, and diagnostic reasoning, *problem solving* is the most commonly used.

It is unfortunate that, in medicine, the term implies that the task of the physician is primarily one of solving problems. Since many medical problems are insoluble, the usual task of the physician is to evaluate or analyze his patient's problems as far as possible or necessary, so that they can be managed effectively. Problem solving also suggests that the intellectual process of finding the solution, as in a puzzle or in a mystery, is the objective or end point to this skill, when the treatment or therapeutic aspects of the process really are the appropriate end point. A great deal of undergraduate teaching incorrectly puts emphasis on diagnosis and differential diagnosis as the appropriate end point in working with patient problems. The term problem solving reinforces this emphasis. The term *medical inquiry* focuses on the data-gathering or evaluative aspect of this process, and the terms *clinical judgment* or *medical decision making* focus on the decision-making component of this process. For these reasons, *clinical reasoning* has been chosen as a term to encompass all the cognitive skills implied in patient evaluation and management. The additional psychomotor skills or techniques of patient interview and physical examination (clinical skills) and the skills or techniques used in diagnostic or treatment procedures are employed by the physician as he exercises his clinical reasoning.

It has been expressed many times that the physician's clinical reasoning process is an "art." Whatever the "good ol' doc" does with the patient is intuitive and not amenable to analysis. If it is considered "intuitive," the implication is that it cannot be taught. Some feel that this process appears only after the physician has had sufficient clinical experience. These opinions are understandable and not entirely incorrect. The steps that occur in the reasoning process of the physician are very rapid and performed almost unconsciously. Several studies have shown that the physician is largely unaware of his own cognitive processes (Barrows & Bennett, 1972; Barrows et al., 1978). In addition, the experienced physician has very facile skills. He can rapidly switch from direct inquiries about the possible nature of the patient's problem to routine screening questions without any observable change in behavior. There is evidence that this reasoning process does not develop in the usual undergraduate and postgraduate educational settings. It begins to surface when the physician enters clinical practice, where he assumes the full pressure of patient responsibility with insufficient time to meet these pressures. This is particularly true if he continues to employ the detailed, comprehensive workups he was taught in his formal education. The pressure of patient responsibility provides impetus to use more time-efficient cognitive processes to evaluate and treat patients. It is unfortunate, however, to give the impression that what the physician does is an art, is intuitive, is not directly teachable, and can occur only with experience. Many students are allowed to become physicians with inappropriate, inaccurate, and inefficient clinical reasoning processes. Unless the cognitive skills a student uses in the clinical reasoning process are appropriately evaluated by relevant techniques, this inadequacy may never be noted (Barrows & Bennett, 1972; McGuire, 1972). Since tools relevant to evaluating the clinical reasoning process are rarely used, no one knows to what extent shoddy clinical reasoning skills may have contributed to inadequate evaluation or treatment of patients. Given the vagaries of patient response and compliance, even imposters can do well in medicine as long as they have a "professional" manner.

Misunderstanding of the physician's clinical reasoning has also resulted from many well-intentioned but inaccurate attempts to characterize this process through introspection. Successful clinicians, usually academic physicians, wish to provide their students with a scheme or structure to approach the evaluation and management of patients. They present to their students an approach that they think is based on the cognitive techniques that they have developed over their years of experience. Not only is this personal introspection dangerously inaccurate as a method for studying cognitive process, it also seems to be distorted by the physician's desire to appear orderly or "scientific." To rearrange your cognitive steps to fit the acceptable medical "norm" is not unlike tidying up the house for company so that they will think you are a good housekeeper. Both Medawar (1969) and Einstein (quoted in Medawar) have accused scientists of this distortion in their introspections. Elstein et al. (1972) have referred to this as the "traditional medical lore" that is found in many textbooks of medicine.

Valid insights into the physician's clinical reasoning process have been gained, however, by a few researchers who have been concerned about scientific thinking both in and out of medicine (Medawar, 1969; Campbell, 1976; Bartlett, 1958; Chamberlain, 1965). Over the last decade, a few formal investigations have helped characterize more accurately the various components of the clinical reasoning process (Kleinmuntz, 1968; Elstein et al., 1972, 1978; Barrows & Bennett, 1972; McWhinney, 1972; Barrows et al., 1978; Feightner et al., 1977).

The various recent studies by Barrows, Feightner, Neufeld, & Norman (1978) at McMaster University and by Elstein, Shulman, & Sprafka (1978) at Michigan State University have employed techniques that permit a more accurate analysis of the physician's approach to the patient encounter. The first of these techniques is the simulated patient: a normal person carefully trained to portray accurately a patient's history and physical examination (Barrows, 1971). These simulations are of such accuracy that they can escape detection by experienced clinicians (Burri et al., 1976). This permits the investigators to choose a specific problem for the physician to encounter that is both real and yet standardized; a problem that is unvarying from physician to physician. Most previous studies have not presented an actual patient; rather, information regarding the case was written or spoken by others. The reality of the simulation ensures that the behavior shown by the physician is representative of his behavior with real patients. The standardization of the simulation allows the investigators to analyze the performance of many physicians for the significant common features that they display in their behavior while working with the same problem. Since the information available and the problem presented by the standardized simulation is known in detail, the variations seen in physician performance can be compared to such outcomes as diagnosis or problem formulation, management plans, time required, and patient satisfaction. With the use of standardized simulation the investigators can also determine the effects of different types of patient problems on the physician's performance.

The second technique employed is the "simulated recall." The physician's encounter with the simulated patient is videotaped through one-way glass. Immediately after the encounter, while the experience is still fresh in his mind, the physician is asked to review this videotape. During the interview, he is carefully questioned in a nondirective manner as to his thinking throughout the encounter. The videotape is stopped at various points to allow for discussion. This can be a potent experience for any clinician. The reliving of an encounter with the patient, while the experience is still fresh, allows the subject to become aware of his thought processes. Many of the physicians who go through this experience find that they realize for the first time how they really think; their processes were unconscious and automatic. (Details of these approaches are available for those who are interested. See Elstein et al., 1972, 1978; Barrows & Bennett, 1972; Barrows et al., 1978.)

The Clinical Reasoning Process

Through the studies just discussed, the nature of the clinical reasoning process and its components has been characterized with considerable specificity. The results obtained from these various investigations over the years tend to support and reinforce each other. The following model has been put together from these sources, as well as with the authors' parallel experiences in observing this process in students, residents, and physicians working with both patients and simulated patients in a variety of educational settings. This model serves as a guide for the design of appropriate educational tools and educational methods to facilitate the evaluation and development of clinical reasoning in students and physicians.

The following descriptions characterize the process in segments that each describe distinctly different behaviors, attempting to put them in a sequence that follows the order of their appearance in the patient encounter.

Step 1

At the onset of his encounter with the patient, the clinician perceives a variety of cues from the patient and the setting in which the patient is encountered. They can be observations about the patient's appearance, age, dress, manner, or movements. They can be taken from the patient's opening remarks, occurring either spontaneously or in response to the physician's own questions. Cues can be taken from information that has come with the patient, such as referral notes; prior records; and comments by parents, spouses, receptionists, or nurses who have accompanied the patient. The particular verbal and nonverbal cues that the physician selects from all this information available in the patient encounter are largely determined by his past patient experiences and the objectives implied by the health-care setting in which the encounter takes place, for example, the emergency room, specialty clinic, hospital ward, or primary care office. The cues he selects are perceived instantly and almost unconsciously. They represent his initial data about the problem and are assembled into an "initial concept" of the problem. This initial concept may be identical to the patient's verbalized complaints and appearance, for example, "a sixtyish, slightly obese man complaining of chest pain." This initial concept may be enriched or modified, however, by cues that may represent a picture different from the patient's verbalization. For example, the physician may be thinking, "a very anxious young lady with multiple complaints," even though the patient may be talking about headache, dizziness, and tiredness. This initial concept, assembled at lightning speed from the cues perceived from the environment, starts the whole direction and scope of the clinical reasoning process.

Step 2

Within moments after the initial encounter, almost simultaneously with the initial concept, the physician generates anywhere from two to five hypotheses that literally pop into his mind as possible explanations for the patient's problem as he has conceived it from his initial concept. This term hypothesis refers to "ideas," "hunches," "guesses," "impressions," and, at times, even "diagnoses" that serve as labels to explain the possible causes for the problem presented by the patient (disorders, diseases, syndromes, organ system dysfunctions, anatomical or physiological derangements, psychological mechanisms, and so on). These hypotheses can be as broad and vague as "something wrong with the heart" or as focused and specific as "thrombosis of the left middle cerebral artery." The collection of hypotheses serves as the guide for the physician's interview and examination of the patient. They represent the initial possibilities that he feels need to be pursued and often may represent concerns, particularly in emergency situations, for conditions that are likely and treatable. They are based on the very little initial data picked up from the cues described previously. All the working hypotheses that the clinician will use are usually developed within the first quarter of his encounter with the patient. They are critical to his clinical reasoning because they are the guide to his inquiry and examination of the patient.

These hypotheses are usually a product of the clinician's past experiences with patient problems. Their appearance from the physician's memory banks is largely an unconscious act of memory association. Many clinicians are unaware of the existence of these hypotheses in their thinking and will say that they had no initial ideas about the cause of the patient's problem, yet the videotape shows that they immediately began asking the patient a chain of specific questions that were obviously based on concerns for a particular disorder, disease, or organ system dysfunction. When asked why these questions were asked, the clinician invariably will describe two or more "hypotheses" he actually was considering all along. It is the automatic or unconscious nature of this process that has made it difficult for physicians to realize how they actually think. The specific questions he asks of the patient and the items of physical examination he performs are, for the most part, specifically chosen to rule in or rule out, or strengthen or weaken, the likelihood of several hypotheses he has entertained in his mind. There may be a tendency for physicians to start with broad or vague hypotheses and to make them progressively more specific and focused as more data is obtained in the encounter. The generation of multiple hypotheses is the creative part of the reasoning process where unusual, novel, or more accurate possibilities for the patient's problem can be thought of as tentative guides to the clinician's search.

In this process, the multiple hypotheses are processed in parallel form, not sequentially. Parallel processing is a more efficient method for problem solving than gathering data to verify or eliminate one hypothesis at a time. Also, the multiplicity of the hypotheses prevents the clinician from prematurely concluding or closing on an obvious but possibly incorrect hypothesis or diagnosis, or from being biased by a favorite hypothesis. Multiple cooperative causes for the problem are more likely to be found when many hypotheses are generated. The effectiveness of considering multiple hypotheses has been well described, and justified for scientific thinking in general, by Bartlett (1958) and Chamberlain (1965).

Step 3

The physician acquires information to shape or refine his early hypotheses by using a variety of data-collection techniques, particularly interview and physical examination. In doing this he attempts to verify hypotheses or, if that is not possible, to rank them in order of likelihood. Much of the clinician's inquiry in this segment of the process can be characterized best as a "search and scan" approach. The questions he asks to establish, shape, refine, strengthen, or rule out his hypotheses are "search" questions, deliberately asked to deduce which of the ideas or hypotheses he has in his head are most likely responsible for the problem presented by the patient. In comparison to the creativity of hypothesis generation, this deductive process requires a rigorous concern for choosing inquiries that will best yield an answer and for carefully analyzing the value of the data obtained in supporting or denying hypotheses. The experienced clinician is efficient in this search; his questions or examinations usually are chosen to produce data that relate to at least two or more of his hypotheses at once.

When the physician comes to a blind alley in his questioning, that is when he is unable to further rank, verify, deny, or refine hypotheses, he switches to "scan" questions for new cues or data that might change his concept or formulation of the patient's problem or the hypotheses he has in his mind. This scan is usually in the form of "functional inquiries" or a "review of systems," questions about common symptoms of various organ systems, and questions about the patient's background and medical history. Routine items on the physical examination also represent scanning. When a new cue that seems relevant or important appears from scans, a new hypothesis or a shift in the order of his present group of hypotheses may occur and a search for new data based on these expanded or revised hypotheses is undertaken.

Routine or scan questions play a minor role in his clinical reasoning process. One of the most prevalent myths about the clinical reasoning process is the belief held by many physicians that comprehensive data gathering, unrelated to specific hypotheses, is an important feature of the clinical reasoning process. Unfortunately, generations of medical students have been carefully trained to take complete and comprehensive history and physical inventories in the fear that they might miss something. Experienced clinicians, who should know better, insist that they use comprehensive assessments, unbiased by initial diagnostic ideas. An experience with a videotaped recall of their own patient encounter has a remarkable effect on these clinicians. They often are ashamed or shocked to realize how problem-oriented they really are in their approach to the patient. Some even express the concern that medical students not see their videotape, since this is not what students have been taught! Logic alone should suggest that the clinician's data-gathering process has to be relevant to what he perceives is the patient's problem, or hours might be spent gathering data of low value. Even worse, if the clinician does not have a good idea as to what might be wrong with the patient, he may not even perceive or attempt to perceive significant data if it appears in front of him. A clinician can completely deny that a certain answer was given by the patient or certain findings were elicited on physical examination when the data did not relate to any of the ideas or hypotheses in his mind (Kleinmuntz, 1968; Barrows & Bennett, 1972).

Although scanning is not the major activity in the patient encounter, it is used to (1) look for new cues that might indicate some aspect of the problem that was overlooked, (2) fill in background data, (3) satisfy the needs of more compulsive clinicians, and (4) increase confidence that the decisions made about the patient's problem are correct. It often is used to provide a conversational filler during the interview process, allowing the physician time to think or ponder about the problem the patient presents without the patient being aware of his quandary. The amount of scanning also depends on the time pressures that exist during the encounter.

Not only does the physician employ a problem-oriented search strategy in a well-disciplined, logical approach to the patient, he also employs short-cuts in his inquiry that can effectively increase the efficiency of his investigation. His initial questions often tend to rule in or rule out a large number of possible hypotheses and to limit the patient's problem to a workable size. Kleinmuntz (1968) pointed out that the experienced physician uses such "maximization principles" in his search. These are "rules of thumb" or heuristics that have high payoff in sorting out the possible causes of certain patient problems. In his study, the more experienced physicians came to correct conclusions about the patient using the least number of questions. The experienced clinician or neurologist in his study had learned to search his problem environment for those symptoms and signs that yielded the greatest amount of data. Such a strategy allowed the physician to radically reduce his problem area or space with a few choice questions. De Dombal (1972) also describes the usefulness of these "maximization principles" in what he calls "algorhythms," which are standard approaches to certain problems that greatly reduce the number of moves that are necessary in problem solving. This is necessary in any game situation where certain initial moves tend to reduce the possibilities to a workable size. Physicians tend to have such "rules of thumb" for a variety of presenting patient problems (Leaper et al., 1973). Such shortcuts, used by primary-care physicians where efficient time utilization is crucial, have often been looked upon by specialists, particularly in academic settings where there is less time constraint, as evidence of sloppy or shoddy thinking. Mechanic & Parson (1975) stress this point in their article, "Short Cuts Are Not Necessarily Bad."

The physical examination seems to be used by the clinician to confirm any hypotheses that still remain likely after he has completed the interview. Although more ritualistic and mechanical than the history, it is still used in a problem-oriented or search approach. The clinician usually knows exactly what he is going to look for when he starts his physical examination of the patient and is usually confident about what he expects to find. Sometimes the clinician does not expect to find anything, but performs an examination because he feels it is expected by the patient. Some physicians rather liberally mix physical examination and history together. In many cases, a positive finding on physical examination, for example, an elevated blood pressure in a patient with morning headaches, can save time in the interview and make the history more productive and focused.

The choice of laboratory tests, diagnostic procedures, and consultations are also an integral part of this inquiry strategy. It occurs to many physicians, usually in the middle of their questioning and examination procedures, that there is a need for certain tests to sort out their hypotheses. Because of the time involved in obtaining data from these tests, compared to the immediacy of the information that can be obtained from questioning and examining the patient, tests are selected as an extended evaluation incorporated into the overall management plan for the patient's problem. Requests for a "battery" of tests may represent both search and scan concerns blended together, but this procedure is not part of an efficient inquiry strategy because of delayed feedback. The medical-legal significance attached to many tests, as well as expected routines for tests in many clinical settings, also affect the clinician's inquiry strategy.

The degree to which this data-gathering endeavor is problem-oriented can be seen from the recent study of Barrows et al. (1978). In their study of 62 physician encounters by physicians randomly selected for study, they found that 61 percent of the physicians' questions were search questions. Almost 75 percent of all the significant information about the patient available on interview was obtained by the physicians before the encounter was half finished. Practically all the hypotheses used in the entire encounter appeared within the first quarter of the encounter (average encounter time was 30 minutes). On the average, physicians in this study obtained only 66 percent of the available information from the patient that could have been helpful in evaluating and managing his problem. This had no effect on the accuracy of the physicians' eventual diagnosis or management. In other words, the physicians could have spent another hour or more obtaining more information, possibly pushing the yield of significant data to 100 percent, without increasing their effectiveness but certainly decreasing their efficiency!

The physician's inquiry strategy employs the psychomotor or clinical skills of interview and examination. In this activity he is guided by hypotheses to select a strategic sequence of inquiries designed to ferret out data that will deduce, verify, deny, focus, or rank the hypotheses in his head in the most efficient and effective manner possible.

Step 4

As the encounter with the patient progresses and the physician elicits more and more information in his search and scan endeavors, a large amount of information accumulates. Even though a small amount of the information obtained may be felt to be relevant to his hypotheses and can support some and weaken others, the total amount of significant information the clinician needs to remember becomes large. This quantity of data elicited cannot be retained in the working memory along with the hypotheses being considered unless it is organized or condensed into some memorable form. The mechanism the clinician seems to employ is to add all the new data he perceives as significant during the encounter to his "initial concept," which has been synthesized from the initial cues he perceived at the beginning of the encounter. As this data is added, a growing or evolving picture of the patient is produced, a "formulation" of the patient's problem that at any given time in the encounter encapsulizes the significant information obtained since the initial cues. [Kassirer et al. (1978) suggest the term "case building" for this behavior.] The resulting formulation also includes significant negative data: information that should have been found on the basis of hypotheses entertained but was not present. This process of problem formulation can be seen in experienced physicians as they communicate to each other about a patient problem. They use brief sentences that often represent an encapsulation or distillation of hours or days of investigation. If you interrupt an experienced clinician during a patient encounter and ask him about the patient, he inevitably will produce just such a concise formulation, with little or no hesitation. This is seen repeatedly in the research done on physicians. During their stimulated recall, they frequently and spontaneously verbalize a concise summary of how they envisioned the patient's picture at various times during the encounter. Again, this is mostly an unconscious activity on the part of the physician. It is the absence of a problem formulation that causes students to recite endless amounts of data about findings on the history and physical examination of a patient when asked for a summary of the patient's problem. This behavior characteristically produces marked discomfort for supervising clinical faculty, since they do not get a clear picture of the patient's problem from the student's presentation. It is remarkable how much more effective students become in their clinical reasoning process when they are required to present a clear, concise, ongoing problem formulation during their patient inquiry.

In conceptualizing these segments as a model for the clinical reasoning process, it is important to realize how dynamic the process is, making it almost impossible to describe adequately in the linear format of words. Significant data or cues gained from search or scan can modify the problem formulation, alter hypotheses, change the ranking of hypotheses, and create new ones. This in turn leads to a different search in other areas, producing new information; so the process continues.

Step 5

At some point in the encounter, the clinician makes a decision that he has obtained all the data he needs or all the information that is available at the time, or decides that no more information is going to help in his concerns about the patient, or decides that the patient's problem is urgent and that immediate care or treatment is needed. If it is not an emergency, this point of "closure" is not a crucial factor and the length of his work with the patient may reflect the time available. In the study by Barrows et al. (1978), the physicians studied chose the hypotheses most likely to explain the patient's problem and obtained most of the significant information about the patient in the first ten minutes of the encounter. Although the physicians' evaluation went on for 30 or more minutes, they could have easily been stopped in 10 minutes with no adverse effect on the accuracy of their diagnostic decision. Considerable time in the encounter is spent in a variety of areas, including (1) scanning to be sure that data has not been overlooked and to gain more confidence in the hypotheses chosen, (2) making additional inquiries to get to know the patient as a person, (3) asking questions that are helpful in selecting treatment or management options, and (4) asking questions about the convenience of hospitalization, willingness to have investigations, other medications the patient may be taking or prior reactions to medications. This half of the encounter was also used to build patient confidence, by asking about concerns the patient might have and their understanding of the problem, and for communicating to the patient about the physician's impressions of the problem and plans for investigations and treatment.

In an emergency situation, such as coma or an acute anginal attack, the clinical reasoning process is abbreviated. This setting represents a challenge for an efficient and effective clinical reasoning process. The physician immediately assesses initial cues and gathers only the data that has the highest priorities and payoffs in terms of evaluating and managing possible life-threatening problems. The hypotheses or diagnoses that the clinician uses are selected more on their usefulness in deciding how the patient's problem is to be managed with maximum payoff. His interventions are aimed at the most life-threatening and most probable causes for the problem.

In many patient encounters, clinicians never come to anything as refined as a diagnosis. Their hypotheses are usually only as accurate as the data obtained allows and serve as an effective guide for further investigations, management, and follow-up of the patient's problem. It often would be a mistake to come to a diagnostic conclusion that was more specific than the patient data would allow, as the physician's mind may become closed to alternative explanations and investigations of the problem as it develops; therefore, at closure the clinician should have decided on the most likely hypothesis or hypotheses to explain the origins or nature of the patient's problem. Although the hypotheses may not be more refined than "a lesion in the left hemisphere" if the data obtained would not allow for more precision, this is called a "diagnostic decision." At closure, the clinician also has decided if he is going to intervene or not intervene, if he is going to order further tests or consultations and if he is going to treat the patient medically, surgically, or psychologically, and how. This is a "therapeutic decision." Closure represents the decision-making segment of clinical reasoning; the evaluation is finished and the next actions have been decided upon.

The physician uses his notes to increase his memory capacity for items that he feels may be significant, details that he may want to review before he closes, and as an aid to prepare his formal record of the encounter. Sometimes during an encounter he will note a cue, observation, or a concern that he will want to pursue later, as it is not part of his ongoing search strategy at the time. His working notes are particularly valuable in this activity. They certainly represent a personal system that can be incomprehensible to anyone else. With his mental problem formulations, likely hypothesis or hypotheses, and his written notes, he is ready to prepare whatever formal record is required of the particular encounter—consultation note, type of progress note, problem-oriented record, or whatever.

Putting It Together

In all this we have concentrated on only the identifiable and common cognitive steps in the clinician's reasoning activities. This clinical reasoning activity is combined with each physician's personal style, which employs techniques to ensure effective interpersonal rapport and to establish effective communication and compliance. The use of body language, small talk, open-ended questions, probes about attitudes, and encouragement to relate concerns are intermixed in the clinical reasoning process. This adds personal "art" to the "science" of clinical reasoning. One of the most fascinating aspects of this art is the way physicians adapt their approach and manner to their perception of the personality, needs, and expectations of the particular patient. This is "acting" in every sense of the word and shows a sensitivity to the human elements of the evaluation process.

Again, it is no small wonder that many observers thought that the physician's approach to the patient was an intuitive art, not a science, and incapable of description. His external behaviors and the sequence of questions and examinations performed give no clue to the reasoning process in his head. He switches from search to scan. He employs maximization strategies. He switches from evaluative actions to actions performed solely to enhance interpersonal communication. He tests multiple ideas in parallel. He performs some actions while taking the history and giving the physical that just buy him time to think or entertain the patient. Once the process is understood, as revealed by contemporary studies, a third-party observer can gain an appreciation of the physician's approach. Once this clinical reasoning process is understood by clinicians, they often become aware of many aspects of their own performance of which they were previously unaware, such as their almost instantaneous and unconscious cue perception and hypothesis formation. Having externalized their own process, they are in a better position to facilitate its development in students. Most clinicians feel that this model fits with the way they perform.

The following table is an edited and abbreviated excerpt from the first minutes of a videotaped, stimulated recall of a physician encounter with a patient. It demonstrates many of these segments of the clinical reasoning process in action. The physician's thoughts in quotation marks are the evolving problem formulation and the thoughts preceded by question marks are hypotheses. Keep in mind that the physician's inquiries and the patient's answers were far more elaborate and natural than shown here.

Table 2-1.

Physician's questions	Patient's answers	Physical examination	Physician's thoughts on recall
He introduces himself	Patient responds		
Name?	Answers		"Old man, appearing short of breath, sitting forward . . .
Age?	67		
How long have you been short of breath?	Since 11:00 A.M. yesterday		? Congestive failure ? Pneumothorax ? Pulmonary embolus ? Coronary
Was it sudden?	Yes		"Old man, short of breath, sitting forward, sudden onset . . .
			? Arrythmia
Were you doing something?	Sawing wood	Takes pulse	"Old man, short of breath, sitting forward, sudden onset, steady pulse . . .
Do you have pain as well?	Yes		? Air embolism ? Pneumothorax

(continued)

Table 2-1. *(continued)*

Physician's questions	Patient's answers	Physical examination	Physician's thoughts on recall
What does it feel like?	Dull ache behind breast bone	Listens to chest	"Old man, short of breath, sitting forward, sudden onset, steady pulse, with substernal pain and good breath sounds . . .
Has it been constant?	Fluctuates	Takes blood pressure	"Old man, short of breath, sitting forward, sudden onset, steady pulse, with substernal pain and good breath sounds, normal blood pressure . . .
Is sitting comfortable?	Any change aggravates pain		? Pericarditis
What if you lie down?	Worse	Listens to heart	"Old man, short of breath, sitting forward, sudden onset, steady pulse, with substernal pain and good breath sounds, normal blood pressure, no rub . . .
Pain in one spot or does it radiate?	One spot		? Gastrointestinal problem
			"Old man, short of breath, sitting forward, sudden onset, steady pulse, with substernal pain and good breath sounds, normal blood pressure, no rub, non-radiating pain . . .

(continued)

Table 2-1. *(continued)*

Physician's questions	Patient's answers	Physical examination	Physician's thoughts on recall
Anything like this before?	Two months ago		"Old man, short of breath, sitting forward, sudden onset, steady pulse, with substernal pain and good breath sounds, normal blood pressure, no rub, non-radiating pain, had prior attack . . .
Tell me about it?	Gradual onset over 10 minutes		? myocardial infarction (must be ruled out will plan to admit to hospital)
	(Interview continues in similar manner.)		

Opposing Points of View

There are many who will deny that the approach just described is either correct or appropriate. They insist that the student should not or cannot form early hypotheses to focus the investigation of the patient. Instead, they feel that the student should ask all the important questions and perform all the important examinations in an unbiased manner. When the student is finished he should then evaluate the data and synthesize it into a diagnosis and differential diagnosis. We think this approach is illogical from the outset, as the student could spend days asking the patient all the questions that are possible and performing a complete examination.

How can the student determine what questions or examinations are important unless he has an idea (or ideas) about the patient's problem? Anyone dealing with a patient must make some decisions about the problem at the very beginning, just to contain the exercise within reasonable proportions from the standpoint of time and effort alone. No clinician would do an extensive inquiry and examination of the back on someone who has no back complaints but who is suffering from progressive dementia; nor would they perform a detailed abdominal examination on someone who appears well and is complaining of an earache. In addition, logic alone would indicate that the clinician could not arrive at a final or appropriate path by starting off the investigation in any direction. The physician must have some idea of where he is going. The investigations of the clinical reasoning process indicate that the student not only should have *some* idea, he ought to have a *good* idea where he is going in the investigation. His approach must be oriented to a concept of the patient's problem. If the clinician needs some idea about the possible areas involved in the problem, then he may as well approach the problem effectively and efficiently. Too many examples are seen of clinicians or students who cannot pull together a patient's problem, who miss important findings, who fail to see the significance of certain data or cues because their mind is devoid of good working hypotheses or problem formulations. As mentioned before, the greatest irony lies in the fact that studies of many physicians who preach unbiased approaches, emphasizing the need for extensive lists of questions and compulsive examination routines, reveal on formal examination that they do not employ this technique themselves when dealing with patients in their own practice. When their inquiry technique is exposed to careful scrutiny, their approach is the same as that described previously. They do not practice what they preach, with good reason: what they preach does not work!

Possibly the reason that many insist that the student should not depend so heavily on a problem-solving approach but instead should employ comprehensive surveys of questions and examinations is that they do not fully understand the power of good problem solving that makes use of appropriate multiple hypotheses and problem formulations (Platt, 1964; Chamberlain, 1965). Take, for example, the case of an older woman who developed diarrhea. Her physician's investigation lead to examination and biopsy of a prolapsed rectum. The biopsy revealed "colitis" and an appropriate management was offered. Her symptoms continued, so another clinician, utilizing a broader range of hypotheses, pursued enough data during clinical examination to discover the subtle signs of a polyneuropathy, eventually found to be secondary to multiple myeloma and amyloidoses. Ironically, the original biopsy of the prolapsed rectum showed amyloid. *The safety of the physician's skill cannot depend on comprehensive inventories, it must depend upon good skills in hypothetico-deductive reasoning.* In this case, the first physician's hypothesis was probably too limited. Even when a comprehensive survey of the patient's symptoms and signs revealed numbness of the hands and feet, the significance was missed because no hypotheses were being entertained to make that data significant. It is a common experience for clinical preceptors to listen to a student's presentation of a patient history and expect findings, on the basis of the history, that the student claims he did not find. When the perceptor examines the patient, the findings are elicited. This is not because the preceptor's technique is better. It is because he had a hypotheses that focused his examination and sharpened his perceptions.

Confirmation from Work in Artificial Intelligence

A fascinating confirmation of this clinical reasoning process comes from the work of Pauker, Gorry, Kassirer, & Schwartz (1976). They realized that most computer programs that have been used in medical diagnosis or decision making could not produce intelligent behavior as it occurs in "real world" situations. These investigators employed the more sophisticated computer technology used in artificial intelligence research to produce a more realistic simulation of the clinician's behavior and thereby obtain better insights into his cognitive processes. They started with personal introspections and observations of colleague physicians as a basis for an initial computer program. They tested this program by presenting the computer with a series of patient problems that featured edema. They compared the computer's questioning strategy and its subsequent printout of the present illness to the behaviors of physicians working with the same patient problems. By noting discrepancies, they felt they were able to recognize components of the clinician's reasoning process that had been either misunderstood or not seen in their initial analysis. On the basis of these discrepancies, they revised the computer's program and repeated the process. This process apparently was repeated until the computer's program closely simulated the inquiry behavior and presented the same clinical write up produced by the physicians on which it was modeled.

Their description of the computer strategies required to produce this successful result provide a fascinating confirmation of the model synthesized from the formal direct studies of the physician. As there were innumerable facts that the computer could gather about the patient, it was apparent that a focus was needed. To do this, their computer program used the patient's chief complaint to generate early hypotheses about the patient's condition. These hypotheses served as a guide to the computer's inquiry. Hypothesis testing was another operation in the computer program that determined how well each hypothesis generated fit to the case being analyzed. The complexities of this program could rank the hypotheses according to fit and eliminate those that did not fit. The investigators noted that the competence of the present illness program depended critically on the computer's ability to generate hypotheses quickly when only a few isolated facts were available. In its overall operation, the computer's program would alternate between asking questions to gain new information and integrating this information into a developing picture of the patient. Although this brief review does not cover many of the ingenious aspects of this study, it is easy to see a now familiar process: problem-oriented inquiry, early generation of multiple hypotheses as a guide to inquiry, the use of inquiry strategies to define and rank hypotheses, and the generation of a patient problem formulation to manage the data obtained.

Significance to Problem-Based Learning

This chapter has gone into considerable detail in summarizing the evidence that is available to help us understand the skill used by the physician to "evaluate and manage patients with medical problems effectively, efficiently, and humanely." Medical educational programs must prepare their students to be able to undertake this task with professional mastery. This chapter has provided the information that is the basis for the technique, tools, and evaluation procedures described in the remainder of this book. The next chapter will review the model proposed from this information base and the relevant educational issues.

CHAPTER 3

Educational Implications of the Clinical Reasoning Process

In Chapter 2, the information available about the physician's clinical reasoning when confronted with a patient problem was reviewed in some detail. The significant aspects of this process can be summarized as follows.

The physician

1. Perceives initial cues from the patient and environment
2. Rapidly generates multiple hypotheses
3. Applies an inquiry strategy (questions, examinations, tests) to refine, rank, verify, or eliminate these hypotheses
4. Abstracts an enlarging problem formulation from the significant, hypothesis-related data obtained from ongoing inquiry
5. Closes the encounter when he has made diagnostic and/or therapeutic decisions.

This clinical reasoning process can be divided conveniently into the following distinct behaviors that can be evaluated and learned.

1. Information perception and interpretation
2. Hypothesis generation
3. Inquiry strategy and clinical skills
4. Problem formulation
5. Diagnostic and/or therapeutic decisions (closure)

Figures 3-1, 3-2, and 3-3 show the individual segments of the clinical reasoning process and their sequence.

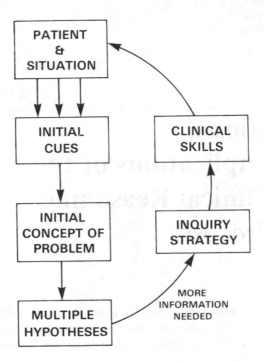

Figure 3-1. The clinician picks up cues from the patient and his setting, forms an initial concept of the problem, and instantly generates multiple hypotheses concerning the nature or cause of the problem identified. Since more information always is necessary at this point, he embarks on a strategy of inquiry, employing his clinical skills to obtain relevant information from the patient.

Implications of this Process for Education

These segments of the clinical reasoning process occur very rapidly in the mind and their actual presence often is unrecognized. In order to help any student develop his intuitive or native problem-solving ability into an effective, efficient clinical reasoning process, these segments of the process must be brought into awareness so that they can be evaluated and appropriate practice and study can improve their quality. Problem-based learning permits these segments of the cognitive process involved in clinical reasoning to be made visible to both student and teacher so they can be modified or developed. To this end, the following discussion is an amplification of each of the identified segments in the process just described. It attempts to review the thinking challenges presented to the student in each of these segments, the

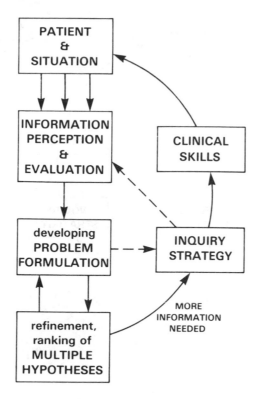

Figure 3-2. More information is perceived as a result of his actions. This information is evaluated and the significant bits are added to his initial concept. The significant information is that which is deemed relevant to his needs to establish, refine, or rank the possible hypotheses in his head. The initial concept grows, by virtue of this information, into an evolving formulation of the problem. This circular process repeats itself during a problem-oriented search for the data necessary to evaluate and manage the patient's problem.

tools or techniques that are helpful in their development, and areas in which a poor performance can have an effect on the entire reasoning process.

Information Perception and Interpretation

Important information of all varieties is available from the very beginning of the clinician's encounter with the patient. The patient's age, sex, dress, manner, and speech all can be perceived. Certain expectations based on experiences gained from previous contact with patients usually determines what information is perceived and abstracted, from this wealth of information, into

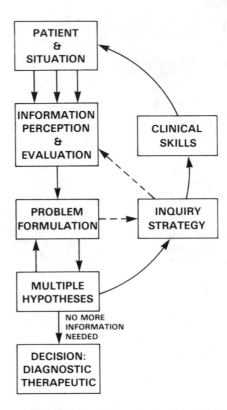

Figure 3-3. When the clinician has obtained sufficient information to establish his hypothesis or probable hypotheses, he closes the process and makes diagnostic and management decisions (please refer to the text for more details).

an initial concept of the problem the patient presents. Some information can precede the contact with the patient, such as referral letters or verbal descriptions of the patient by someone who saw him previously. It is important that students discipline themselves to be consciously aware of all the information available and to consider how it could be useful in identifying the patient's problem or problems. As the patient begins the encounter by giving his story, more valuable information can be perceived. Information should include not only the possible medical problems but the patient's personality, emotions, concerns, reactions to the physician, level of intelligence, level of consciousness, and his ability to communicate. The patient's response to questions from the physician continues to produce more valuable information. Considering the great amount of information that issues from any patient, it is apparent that a management system is necessary for the clinician to retain and evaluate the important data that is produced. The concern in this stage of the process is how much of this potentially valuable information is actually perceived and how accurately is it perceived.

Certainly, the human senses are limited by the scope of the information they can receive; however, the information that is received through the limited apertures of our senses is impressive, far more than we utilize in the average interpersonal interaction. The human mind further reduces and abstracts the information that does come through its senses, through perception or input processing. The physician's perception of the patient can be colored by preconceptions based on past experiences and learning. The information from the patient has to pass through the filters of interpretation and biases in the mind of the clinician. Much of this may be unconscious, learned behavior; many of the past facts and experiences that have shaped these preconceptions are forgotten. Tired housewives, "hippy" adolescents, aggressive businessmen, and complaining mothers are examples of stereotypes that can bias perception consciously or unconsciously. Another filter through which information passes is the clinician's level of attention. If he is tired, somnolent, bored, distracted, or preoccupied, much of the relevant information available may not be perceived.

Arnheim (1969) has shown that visual perception is a very active process. Often, the clinician has to look directly at something and seek it if he is to see it. If you look at one word in the center of this page and fix your eyes there and do not move them, you will notice that you are unable to make out more than a few other words. A graph made of the changing eye directions of one person looking at an object or photograph show clearly that the eyes move around to many areas that seem important, in order to assemble an impression of the object. The perception of the whole is a synthesis in the mind of all these areas on which the vision was fixed. Luria (1973) has suggested that the aphasic patient who cannot recognize or name an object is unable to remember, after his eyes have moved to another point, the previous image from his last fixation on another area of the object. The same phenomenon of focused attention is true for hearing. You hear what you select to hear: an instrument out of the orchestral sound, a voice in a crowd, an idea or phrase in a conversation, or a word or expression from the patient. This focus holds true for all sensory perception. Until you read this sentence, you were probably unaware of the pressure of the belt around your waist, the shoes on your feet or the watch on your wrist. The information carried to our brain is so rich that the mind must focus its perception, consciously or unconsciously.

Perception of data from the patient is an active process and not passive; it is a result of attention, prior conditioning, and conscious search for information. It is clear, therefore, that the initial cues received from the patient, which serve as a stimulus for the physician's hypotheses, represent a crucial step in the quality of the reasoning process. The challenge for the student is to be consciously aware of what information he needs from the patient and his environment. In addition, the student must develop an awareness of how his conscious or unconscious attitudes, interpretations, and biases about the patient or his problem, based on past experiences or beliefs, may alter the picture of the patient problem confronting him.

A closely related problem that can affect the accuracy of this segment of the process is "translation errors." These occur when a patient's symptom or complaints are translated into a medical term in the mind of the clinician, without a careful consideration as to what unwarranted assumptions may have been made. A classic example is the complaint of being "dizzy." The clinician may unquestioningly interpret this as "vertigo"; his hypotheses and subsequent reasoning will be aimed at disentangling possible causes of vertigo. Actually, the patient may have used the word to describe a swimming sensation in the head, unsteadiness, or syncopal feelings. Each meaning has clearly different pathological mechanisms. The clinician may expend a considerable amount of time pursuing the wrong track before it is apparent that vertigo was not a correct translation for the patient's complaint. Worse yet, it may never actually become apparent to the examiner, further reducing the effectiveness of his skills. The student must always dissect or question the complaint of the patient until he is certain what the patient experienced. The student must not apply a premature and possibly incorrect translation using a convenient or short medical term.

The clinician must be concerned about the reliability of information perceived or selected. He may need to elicit, repeatedly and in different ways, the same items of information that may be critical to his reasoning, or he may need to check the reliability of the information. A commonly employed technique is to find external verification for a symptom or complaint by asking a relative or co-worker about the patient's behavior or the consequences of the complaint. For example, a testimony to the severity of a headache as a complaint is whether the patient leaves work to rest in a quiet, dark room or goes to a hospital emergency room for medication.

Hypothesis Generation

Elstein et al. (1972) describe the previous segment by saying that the physician "attends" to the initially available cues from the patient and then almost simultaneously identifies the "problematic elements" from these cues, which then serve as "indexing keys" for long-term memory; as a result, he generates hypotheses as suggestions for further inquiry. He points out that, in any situation in which the problem solver is working in an "open system" in which a number of solutions, resolutions or conclusions are possible, the problem solver must begin from a given starting point and move to a number of possible terminal points. He suggests that scientists, managers, chess players, physicians and many others face this open-ended problem situation every day. This early generation of multiple hypotheses represents a technique for dealing with the problem of reasoning with an open system by transforming that system into a series of hypothetical closed systems, each with a terminal point represented by a hypothesis. The problem solver can then proceed with an inquiry that tests the appropriateness of the proposed end points (Elstein et al., 1972). Certainly, all studies of the physician amply demonstrate his early generation of multiple hypotheses after receiving only a few initial cues or items of patient data. Platt (1964) suggests that better strides are made in scientific investigations when scientists use "strong inference," which he defines, in part, as the creation of multiple hypotheses and the use of experiments to evaluate each hypothesis as a possible outcome. The physician's "experiment" is his inquiry strategy, utilizing clinical skills.

The initial cues that form the initial concept of the patient's problem can affect the generation of hypotheses. For example, if the initial formulation of the problem is "an anxious young girl with acute paralysis of the legs," hypotheses might appear in the clinician's mind, such as conversion hysteria, transverse myelitis, or an extradural spinal cord mass. If the initial data from this girl produced a different initial formulation, such as "a young girl with a slowly progressive paralysis," a totally different set of hypotheses would probably have popped into a clinician's mind, such as epidural tumor, metabolic or degenerative disease of the spinal cord, or congenital or hereditary spinal cord afflictions. If the patient in the emergency room were a middle-aged man with sudden paraplegia, the clinician might consider transverse myelitis, metastases to the spinal cord, and vascular occlusion in the cord, among other hypotheses. These initial hypotheses are generated from the cues that form the patient's initial picture. They provide a guide for further inquiry.

The word hypothesis can be defined as a proposition set forth as an explanation for the occurrence of some specified group of phenomena, merely as a provisional conjecture to guide investigation. In clinical investigation, the term refers to ideas, diagnoses, guesses, models, concepts, candidates, or whatever you may wish to call them, that label possible or proposed explanations that will guide the investigation into the patient's problem.

These hypotheses have many facets that may fall under a variety of subject classifications, depending upon the formulation of the problem in the clinician's mind, his knowledge about medical disease, and his experiences with similar problems. These hypotheses can be syndromes, specific disease entities, disorders (seizures, collagen disease, hypertension), pathological processes (meningitis, cerebrovascular disease, immunological disease), anatomical locations (middle-ear disease, right posterior fossa lesion), or biochemical or physiological derangements (inappropriate antidiuretic hormone secretion, hyponatremia). The hypotheses also vary widely in their specificity, some being very vague and broad and others focused and precise. Some hypotheses have multiple aspects that allow them to be useful across several categories at once. An example is "transverse myelitis," which may imply an anatomical localization, a clinical syndrome, or a group of pathological processes. The degree to which the hypotheses become specific in the physician's mind is usually related to his prior experiences with this category of problem and the specificity that is necessary to select the most appropriate management plan. In everyday clinical use, the "diagnosis" is not the end point of the encounter. The management of the patient's problem or problems is the end point, and hypotheses serve as the needed guide. If no alternative therapeutic advantages are achieved by a more specific diagnosis, it usually is not made. If a too-specific diagnosis is made in the encounter, before laboratory tests or investigations are requested, possible alternatives for the patient's problem may not be sought. The hypotheses should be no more specific than required for management or further investigation.

The generation of hypotheses is often an automatic, learned process. It represents the creative aspect of the problem-solving process. The efficiency, effectiveness, and quality of the clinician's evaluation are largely dependent on the hypotheses generated (Barrows et al., 1978). The development of hypotheses can be seen as parallel to "brain storming" and lateral or divergent thinking. Basically, the richness of the hypotheses produced by the clinician is a product of prior experience and memory, as shown in Figure 3-4. The number and quality of hypotheses can be improved by creating as many as possible for the problem and being concerned about their specificity and appropriateness. It is through this creative aspect of hypothesis generation that innovative, more adequate ways to explain unusual patient problems may be found, or explanations for common, poorly understood problems may be discovered.

If the hypotheses in the clinician's mind are well designed, all the information from the patient should relate to at least one or more of the hypotheses and, therefore, either support or weaken their likelihood as possible causes or explanations for the problem. As mentioned previously, several studies have shown that information elicited from a patient that does not directly relate to any of the clinician's hypotheses usually is forgotten (Kleinmuntz, 1968; Barrows & Bennett, 1972). As there is so much information coming from the patient that needs to be integrated or organized, the student must keep on the alert for data that does not seem to fit any of his hy-

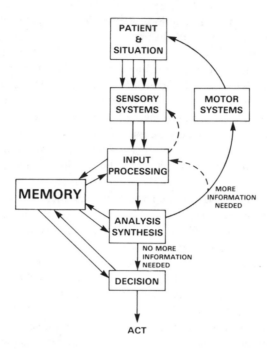

Figure 3-4. This flow chart indicates the important cognitive events in the clinical reasoning process and complements the structures in the previous three figures. It shows that the clinician's sensory systems filter information from the patient and his setting and that the clinician's past experiences and learning filter it even further. Much of this activity is unconscious. The information base from the patient can become reduced or biased prior to synthesis into an abstraction of the patient's problem. "Motor systems" refers to the patterns of muscle contractions used to ask, look, examine, order tests, and so forth. The small arrows indicate that a conscious awareness of the information being perceived or processed can enlarge the available pool of relevant information. Most important, this indicates the crucial role of memory in the effectiveness of the clinical reasoning process and shows how the process itself enriches the memory bank.

potheses. When this occurs, he must challenge either the reliability of that item of data or the adequacy of his hypotheses, and act accordingly. The experienced clinician is seen to create a "net" of hypotheses that will relate in one way or another to almost all the data that may come from a patient with the type of problem presented. In many instances the experienced clinician can be seen to start with broad, generalized hypotheses and, as information unfolds from the patient as a result of his inquiry, to focus or increase the specificity of the more appropriate hypotheses. A very specific hypothesis early in the patient interaction, such as "an embolus in the territory of the middle cerebral artery," might prevent the examiner from appreciating or seeking an explanation for the patient's complaint of cough and weight loss. A broad hypothesis, such as "something wrong in the left hemisphere," might allow the patient's complaint of cough and weight loss to lead to a hypothesis concerning metastases to the brain. Hypotheses that are too specific at the outset may bias the clinician's thinking in a manner that will permit obvious cues from the patient to pass unnoticed; therefore, hypotheses should be made more specific only as more data unfolds from the search as supporting or denying evidence and as is warranted by therapeutic decisions or further investigation.

Multiple hypotheses provide the best insurance that the clinician will not come to a premature decision about the patient's problem, since they force him to consider possible alternative explanations. It has been suggested that the penchant some clinicians have for seeking "rare birds" or unusual diagnoses is a helpful mechanism to prevent such premature closure (Elstein et al., 1972). The number of hypotheses produced usually seems to be more than three and never more than seven. This may relate to the work of Miller (1956), which suggests that the human memory can hold approximately seven "chunks" of information at one time. If the physician needs to entertain more hypotheses, he chunks several hypotheses together into a single hypothesis that labels them in a higher order of abstraction. For example, lupus erythematous and polyarteritis might be lumped together as collagen or immunological disease.

Sets of hypotheses may come in several sequences during the encounter. In neurological problems, it seems probable that the clinician initially entertains hypotheses of anatomical localization. Once the location is established, the neurologist entertains hypotheses concerning etiology, deranged physiology, or the pathological process as present.

As a result, there are many aspects in generating hypotheses that the student needs to consider consciously, oftentimes with faculty guidance, so that this rapid, unconscious process will be creative and most effective in clinical reasoning. They are as follows.

1. Early generation on initial cues
2. Sufficient number and variety of hypotheses to ensure all data are encompassed
3. Conscious consideration, on reviewing the initial cues present, of possible hypotheses that should have occurred automatically but did not
4. Using initially broad, generalized, or anatomical hypotheses until the data allows for more focused concerns.

As a further refinement in hypothesis generation, the experienced clinician may rank likely hypotheses from the standpoint of their life-threatening importance for the patient or of their treatability. It does little good to dwell on a benign possibility or an untreatable condition if serious possibilities or treatable conditions could exist. It is important for the student also to consider priorities for his hypotheses in terms of "payoff." The objective of the patient encounter is to uncover a possible and effective means of reducing, correcting, or minimizing the problem or of avoiding further complications.

Initially, students may be concerned that they do not have sufficient experience or an adequate knowledge base to develop multiple hypotheses when confronted with a patient problem. It has usually been our experience, however, that if students are asked to deliberately think creatively about possible hypotheses, to free-associate about conceivable explanations for the problem, they will come up with workable hypotheses. Even before they enter medical school they have accumulated considerable information about medicine that allows them to develop a number of hypotheses about any patient problem. As they continue to work with more problems, especially in the problem-oriented learning system described in this book, they accumulate more information that enriches their usable knowledge or experience base. This, in turn, will permit more numerous and effective hypotheses to be produced in the future. This is the objective of problem-based learning. It provides the physician with associations in his long-term memory that will facilitate the generation of immediate hypotheses, making him more effective in his reasoning (Figure 3-4). In the beginning, the student may produce only one or two hypotheses to process. They may be incorrect and lead him into a blind alley. He must then "scan" for more cues and more information, and suggest new ideas or hypotheses. Often, the beginning student does not have sufficient knowledge to determine which of his hypotheses is most likely. As will be seen later, this can be a most effective point for the student to stop and study appropriate texts or resources. Repeating this process with patient problems builds up an effective bank of medical data that will make him a most effective clinician.

Inquiry Strategy and Clinical Skills

The term "clinical skills" is usually employed to define the technical or psychomotor skills involved in interview and physical examination, as well as interpersonal or communication skills. The term "inquiry strategy" as used here includes the cognitive processes that select the particular question to be asked and physical examination item to be performed, as well as their sequence. Both are necessary in the clinician's search for information to evaluate the patient's problem, to rank and refine hypotheses, to sharpen the problem formulation and to reach a decision concerning both evaluation and treatment.

The challenge in these segments of the clinical reasoning process is that the clinician's action — that is, his questions on history, items of physical examination, and subsequent choice of laboratory tests or investigations — must be guided by the pool of hypotheses in his mind. The data he searches for and derives must offer direct help by either increasing the likelihood of one or more of the hypotheses in his head or by weakening or ruling out other hypotheses. Ruling out hypotheses is difficult in medicine and physicians have been criticized often for their inability to do this. This may be due to the fact that most disease processes can present with considerable variation in symptoms and signs, in different patients. Many diseases are pleomorphic in their appearance and "formes fruste" of diseases and disorders are common. A hypothesis can be relegated to the position of being unlikely but still can be difficult to eliminate. Appropriate inquiry strategy requires the physician to know what information would be of most value in processing his hypotheses. Elstein et al. (1972) suggested that the excessive use of laboratory tests and investigations occurs when the physician has a group of hypotheses and insufficient amount of significant data available to appropriately rank or verify them. In his strategy of inquiry, the physician has to process his hypotheses in parallel as a more efficient and effective way of achieving appropriate outcomes with a patient problem, so he elicits information important to several hypotheses at the same time. Barrows et al. (1978) have shown that the physician's questions usually relate to two or more of the hypotheses in his mind.

A number of techniques are helpful in this area. First, a conscious effort on the part of the clinician to pick only the actions that would have the highest yield in discriminating among his hypotheses is helpful. Frequently, the rapid, unconscious activities he uses in inquiry may be employed out of habit and not chosen deliberately as being appropriate to the hypotheses generated. Often, clinicians get into an almost mechanical ritual of asking routine questions in certain situations without thinking of their payoff or appropriateness in sorting out the possibilities they have in mind.

A flexibility of style or approach is important, in order to sort out the particular hypotheses regarding the particular patient. There has been a strong emphasis in the training of most physicians to consider the history and the physical examination as two separate parts of the assessment of the patient; however, there are many occasions in which a mixture of history and physical actions would be more efficient. For example, in evaluating a patient with a vague complaint about walking difficulty, observation of the gait early in the encounter may save a lot of time in appropriate inquiry about his problem. There are innumerable instances where an item of physical examination, rather than an answer to a question, may answer more effectively a question relevant to the physician's hypotheses.

There is a large variety of techniques used in the clinical skill of interviewing. They are used both to gain information and to establish a rapport that facilitates the quality and amount of information. Their use is often a personal matter that characterizes the "style" of a particular clinician. The variety of strategies used by individual clinicians can include open-ended questions, forced choices, repetition of the patient's story, silence, and a variety of verbal and nonverbal actions. There are a few basic strategies, however, that are used in both interview and physical examination that reflect the clinician's evaluation of the patient relative to his hypotheses and problem formulations. These were described previously as "search" and "scan" strategies. Search inquiries tend to dissect symptoms as to their subjective quality, their temporal profile, the factors that aggravate or improve them, their association with other symptoms, their effect on the patient, and so forth. They also tend to be focused or aimed at directly seeking specific symptoms or phenomena that would help support, refine, or rank hypotheses.

The physician switches back and forth from search to scan quickly and easily. When his search mode runs into a blind alley or he feels he has gotten all the information he needs or is capable of obtaining at the time, he then scans. Scans are inquiries that are routine data-gathering procedures not related to specific hypotheses. They are necessary to gain background information and to survey other unsuspected areas in which productive cues might be found that are relevant to the problem. Scanning can provide the clinician with time to review the patient's problem in his mind and consider his next actions. It also provides confidence in the evaluation by making certain that nothing else has been missed. The extent of scanning usually depends on the luxury of time available in the encounter and the security of the examiner.

Maximization principles are also important strategies in the efficient approach to problem solving. They reduce the number of questions or actions necessary to come to an understanding of the problem. They represent a series of questions that can rapidly shrink the potential problem to a workable size. These are the shortcuts we all use in a variety of game situations, whether we are playing 20 questions or other such games, or evaluating a patient problem (Kleinmuntz, 1968; de Bono, 1969; Elstein et al., 1972). It is these strategies that have been immortalized in the algorithms that are written for clinician's approaches to standardized problems. These strategic moves or actions are usually learned from prior experiences in working with problems. De Bono pointed out that, after playing a new game for a number of times, players would identify moves and strategies in specific situations that were effective in successful play. Kleinmuntz clearly showed how the use of maximization principles correlated with the clinical experience of the clinicians involved in his study. With something as complex as a patient problem, it's impossible to discover or employ all the possible inquiries that might be useful and to be aware of their potential value in any particular problem. Maximization principles allow the clinician to move more rapidly in narrowing down the possibilities that he has to consider. These maximization principles can be gained by the student from experience with patients and patient simulations in problem-based learning. They also can be learned to some degree from reading the writings of experienced clinicians. To develop and use maximization principles, the student must always review the actions that contributed to his success or difficulty with a patient problem so that these factors can be either developed, modified, or avoided with similar problems in the future.

    Pitfalls in inquiry strategies are the converse of what has been described above. Some clinicians tend to choose their questions or their physical examination items randomly or routinely, without careful thought as to their importance in sorting out their hypotheses. This is a behavior that reduces effectiveness in clinical reasoning. Rigidity in style or approach inhibits the clinician's ability to adapt to the individual differences in patient problems. Sequential processing of one hypothesis after another makes the whole process inefficient and often ineffective. If the clinician begins inquiring from the patient information relevant to only one hypothesis, he not only begins to waste time but he runs the risk of branching the reasoning process, leading himself to a blind alley or even a premature closure on the wrong hypothesis. Parallel processing of multiple hypotheses is crucial; the clinician should make a deliberate attempt to come up with two or more hypotheses in any patient problem and carry out his inquiries relevant to them.

Problem Formulation

Even though the clinician considers or selects only the information he feels is relevant to his hypotheses in his encounter with the patient, this information alone can produce a large body of facts to be kept in his working memory. Combined with the three to seven hypotheses he is considering in his working memory, a system to manage all this accumulated information is needed. Mechanisms are described in cognitive psychology by which one may reduce the amount of information that needs to be carried in what is called the "working memory." As with all the other cognitive mechanisms we have considered, these also can be an automatic and relatively unconscious phenomenon, or they can be deliberate and conscious. Possible mechanisms employed to accomplish this information reduction can be as follows.

1. Retain relevant information only, including relevant negative information. Relevant negative information might concern the absence of a symptom or sign that would be expected with a particular hypothesis that is being entertained. Relevant information is information that helps establish, rank, or rule out hypotheses generated.
2. Retain only the relevant information that has the highest payoff in denying or supporting hypotheses. Although the patient may describe many symptoms or show many signs that can be seen to support a hypothesis, the physician may retain only those few that are required if the hypothesis is to be seriously entertained or others eliminated.
3. Condense information into large chunks by synthesizing, simplifying, or translating it into a term or title that covers its assembled significance (syndromes or disease groups). For example, instead of considering (1) weakness greater in the arm than the leg, (2) increased reflexes, (3) increased tone, and (4) a Babinski sign, the physician lumps it all together as "pyramidal syndrome."
4. Write down on paper any information that conceivably could be needed or important.

During the encounter, the ever enlarging information base about the patient, which is a product of information filtering, reduction, synthesis, and labelling, is formulated into a concise patient story that holds all the data needed to evaluate the hypotheses entertained. This formulation may exist in the clinician's working memory as a visual, verbal, or preverbal abstraction of the patient's problem at any given moment. Elstein et al. (1972) refer to it as the identification of the "problematic element." In the flow charts depicting the clinical reasoning process (Figures 3-1, 3-2, and 3-3), the "formulation" box is derived from the "initial concept" box, which represents the beginning of the patient encounter. This initial concept is developed quickly from the initial cues perceived from the patient and his setting, and stimulates the immediate generation of hypotheses from associations in the clinician's memory. As new information is sought from the patient to refine or rank these hypotheses, the accumulated relative or important information is added in the clinician's mind to this initial concept and it becomes the evolving formulation. The problem formulation is an active, ongoing mental process that represents a summary of the experiences in the encounter to that moment. Its quality can affect the effectiveness of the clinical reasoning process, the generation of hypotheses, the appropriate use of scan and search methods or inquiry strategy, and the refinement of hypotheses.

Good, working problem formulations must include all relevant information, contain no irrelevant or unnecessary information, and be concise. The formulation should not bias hypotheses by containing inaccurate, poorly translated data or by containing overly concise diagnostic labels, particularly labels that represent tacit assumptions. For example, an initial problem formulation such as "this is a fifty-five-year-old depressed man with a left-sided stroke" is concise but it could inhibit appropriate evaluation first by the use of the word "stroke." It is a likely but unwarranted conclusion drawn from the initial information about the patient's problem and may prevent the generation of hypotheses about nonvascular causes of a sudden hemiparesis. Second, the term "depressed" in the formulation could bias hypotheses about the patient's emotional picture, which might not have been due to depression but, instead, to an organic brain syndrome secondary to more diffuse cortical involvement. It would be better to formulate his problem as "this is a fifty-five-year-old man who seems depressed and has a left hemiparesis of sudden onset." In doing this, the clinician has, up to that point in his investigation, provided a formulation that summarizes the problem but will not close his mind to alternatives that could explain the symptomatology. Had he concentrated his inquiry on producing information relevant to the varieties of cerebrovascular disease, because of his formulation with the concept stroke, when indeed the hemiparesis was due to a tumor or generalized metabolic process, he would have been on the wrong track a long time and his reasoning ineffective and inefficient.

The clinician constantly must adapt his formulation to any significant information he obtains from the patient and be certain it is concise, inclusive, and unbiased. As more information is obtained from the patient on interview and examination, the formula may undergo considerable modification and revision as new and sometimes unexpected information appears and hypotheses are changed or refined. This skill in problem formulation requires diligent, conscious practice on the part of the student. As will be seen later, it plays a crucial role in the quality and efficiency of the student's reasoning.

Workers in cognitive psychology have suggested a number of techniques that might be helpful in dealing with a difficult problem that does not seem to be easily resolved or understood by the appropriate application of inquiry skills.

1. *Simplify the problem.* Are there unnecessary elements, symptoms, background data, or other factors present in the patient problem that can be eliminated? In a reverse sense, can the problem be subdivided into subproblems, with one of the subproblems being taken on first to see if it can be understood or resolved? Are there unnecessary relationships, temporal relationships between symptoms and signs, relationships to other disease processes, and so forth, that can be eliminated, allowing the problem to be

considered in a simpler form? The clinician can always expand back to the original problem if this simplification allows him to make progress.

2. *Take a break from the problem.* This usually is accomplished by coming back to the patient after a few moments of private thought, or having the patient make a return appointment. This allows the clinician to let the problem "incubate" and to suspend judgment at that particular time. Many times, creative ideas or new insights into a problem occur at a relatively unconscious level if incubation time is provided.

3. *Force "divergent" thinking.* The clinician should make himself develop a wide variety of hypotheses, no matter how remote some of them might seem. "Brainstorm" hypotheses. This may allow the clinician to see new alternatives that may not have occurred to him before in his approach to the problem.

4. *Alter the manner in which the data is represented.* Examples would be to put down the patient's problem in the form of a diagram or model, drawing relationships of symptoms and signs to events and time. Rearrange the data in the problem; perhaps the laboratory tests ought to be reviewed first or the physical examination data, then the history reconsidered. Rearranging the data often allows new insights to occur in a confusing problem.

5. *Talk the problem out with someone else or present it formally to a group of peers.* Oftentimes when the clinician is forced to express the problem verbally in a manner in which it would be clear enough for someone else to understand, new insights or approaches are gained. In addition, that other person may have some ideas that could have been a blind spot on the part of the clinician, or he may have had an experience or an understanding in the past that will help with the problem.

6. *Find data that can be eliminated.* Get rid of extra data for the time being and work with the residual data.

7. *Try the shortest and most obvious path with the problem.* Even though it may not be totally satisfactory, see where it concludes. This is forcing yourself to use maximization strategies.

8. *Rethink the elements of the problem.* Do this rapidly, forward and backward, up and down, until all the diverse data, perhaps too much to be remembered adequately in the working memory, are finally encompassed in the mind. This may suggest new relationships that have not occurred.

When any problem is particularly difficult, it often is important to review all the elements in the history and physical examination, the hypotheses, and the problem formulation. This review may show that there have been biases or errors in translation that have occurred. It may also show certain tacit assumptions made about the patient problem which may not necessarily be true.

Diagnostic and/or Therapeutic Decisions (Closure)

Although the physician may do his best to verify the most likely hypotheses in his head during his interaction with the patient, many things may operate to prevent this from occuring or even to make this an inappropriate occurrence on a particular occasion. Laboratory studies may be required to provide the data that are essential to sort out hypotheses in the definitive fashion. The opinion of another consultant or a diagnostic investigation may be needed before the hypotheses can be narrowed down or verified. During the encounter, the patient may be fatigued or the problem may seem so complex that more questions and more examinations at that time would yield no further information of any value. The patient's condition may appear urgent and in need of intervention or treatment; even though a specific or refined hypothesis or diagnosis is not possible, action must be taken. All these factors can affect the time it takes a physician to make decisions about the patient's problem and its treatment, thus bringing the encounter to an end.

As shown in the study of physicians' behavior in a half-hour encounter, almost all the necessary information needed to formulate the most likely cause for the problem and decide on management was usually obtained in the first 10 minutes. As mentioned previously this suggests that much time is probably spent in confirming data, searching for other possible cues that have not been identified, establishing rapport with a patient, and gaining confidence in the decisions that were made on the basis of other inquiries. The clinician constantly has to ask himself whether more information is needed, would it be of any benefit if it were obtained, and is it available?

The clinician has a variety of actions that he can take at the point of closure. He can decide, as mentioned above, that he has to act now and intervene with the patient with a management plan, a treatment, or hospitalization. Or, he may decide that there is no hurry and that after some further observation or other tests he may eventually want to intervene with a management plan. Frequently, the physician makes the decision to do nothing; he has evaluated the problem for the time being and has decided nothing needs to be done.

If he decides to intervene, there is a wide variety of actions possible. Many relate to gaining more information, referring the patient for a consultation with another physician or health professional, such as a therapist or a psychologist, or making further laboratory tests or diagnostic investigations. He may decide to treat the patient with medical or pharmacological means, surgical or rehabilitative approaches, or with patient counseling, patient education, or advice.

The ordering of appropriate laboratory investigations or diagnostic studies is another extension of the clinical reasoning process. It produces the data necessary to verify hypotheses and to design an appropriate treatment or management plan. As with all the other segments of the clinical reasoning process, a conscious awareness on the part of the student as to exactly why he is closing and what the appropriate actions to follow should be is a valuable exercise. Closure is the end of only one point in the patient encounter and not an end point itself. The object of the clinical reasoning process is not to verify hypotheses and make a diagnosis and a differential diagnosis. The object is to manage the patient's problem.

Conclusion

The clinical reasoning process is a scientific approach to patient problems. The objective is to be able to evaluate and manage the problems about which the patient or the person referring the patient was concerned. The process has definable segments: perception of initial cues, assembling an initial concept of the problem, generating multiple hypotheses, employing an inquiry strategy, integrating the information elicited into a growing problem formulation, and closing with evaluative and therapeutic decisions. Along with the clinical reasoning process, a number of other concerns are being processed simultaneously in the mind of the skilled physician. All of these concerns are suggested by the following groups of questions.

1. What is this patient's problem; what ideas do I have about its location and cause; what further information do I need; what action shall I take next?
2. Is this problem urgent; should some immediate actions be taken?
3. What sort of a person is this patient; what does the patient expect from me; how is he responding to my approach and personality; should I modify my approach?
4. What is my response to this patient as a person; do I need to watch my reactions? Am I stereotyping him as a personality without good evidence?
5. That was an important piece of information I just learned, but it's not related to the ideas I am pursuing right now; I'll have to hold it and come back to it later.
6. Does this patient have a family or employment problem that may be affecting his complaints or symptoms?
7. I wonder how this patient is going to be managed. Should I prepare the patient for hospitalization during this visit? How well will the patient respond to the idea of a spinal tap?

Although all these concerns may go on in the mind of the experienced clinician, he usually is not aware of the multiple levels of his thinking. It is the ultimate challenge of the student to take on these cognitive activities with confidence and assurance. As simulations help pilots handle the diverse complexities of aircraft, so will the subsequent chapters of this book show how simulation is effective with medical students.

The clinical reasoning process has been discussed in this chapter in considerable detail to provide a basis for details in the subsequent chapters, which describe how it is to be facilitated or developed in the student and how it is to be evaluated. The design of a learning resource aimed at facilitating the development of the clinical reasoning process must take its various components into consideration. Examples of disordered, inefficient, or inaccurate clinical reasoning process seen in medical students and clinicians are described in Chapter 5.

CHAPTER 4

Presenting the
Patient Problem
for Learning

Problem-based learning requires that problems be available for the student to study. They should be in a format that will help him develop his clinical reasoning skills and, at the same time, stimulate appropriate self-directed learning. The components and sequences of the clinical reasoning process that will have to be learned by the student (described in the previous chapter) serve as a guide to the teacher in both the design and use of problems.

Since the majority of problems that the student, as a future physician, will be working with are patient problems, our principle concern in undergraduate medical education should be the presentation of patient problems. Other health problems can be used, however, to meet specific educational objectives that may relate more to public health issues, health administration, health-care delivery systems, and epidemiology. Problems that present themselves in the basic sciences related to medicine also can be used to stimulate critical thinking and appreciation of important biological mechanisms or principles. Some examples of these types of problems will be referred to in the subsequent chapter on the design of problem-based learning units (Chapter 9).

Formats for Presentation

Traditionally, the medical student is presented with patient problems in one of two formats: real patients or written case histories. Each has its particular advantages and disadvantages in the education of the student, all of which should be recognized and considered.

Advantages of Using Real Patients

Nothing can be more motivating for students than to work with real patients. This is the real world of medicine and there is no better way for them to learn than to actually have "hands-on" experience with patients, under the guidance of the teacher. The student's ability to examine, interview, establish rapport, make appropriate observation, and employ all the segments of the clinical reasoning process are exercised. The student can generate hypotheses, employ an inquiry strategy, formulate the problem, evaluate information, and make appropriate decisions. He can see the consequences of his own skill in the data that are acquired; he is challenged to pull it together in a manner that will allow him to identify the patient's problems with sufficient accuracy and devise an appropriate management plan. In addition, work with the real patient allows the student to be progressively introduced to the pressures and responsibilities of patient care.

There is no substitute for learning from real patients, so students must have patient experience from the very first year of medical school. As we describe a variety of learning formats in which patient problems are presented to the student, this point always must be clearly understood. The student always should have the opportunity to transfer into work with patients the knowledge and skills he gains from his studies in problem-based learning. He should be able to apply repeatedly the techniques, skills, and knowledge he has acquired. It is this repeated application of acquired skills and knowledge to new problems that reinforces the use and retention of this knowledge by the student. Its application to real patients also reassures him as to its relevance and importance.

Disadvantages of Using Real Patients

Patient experience often is not the best learning format in which the student can acquire knowledge and clinical skills. The use of patients has a variety of drawbacks if considered from the educational point of view. It may be difficult to accept that there can be better sources of patient problems for learning than actual patients, but the following disadvantages need to be recognized and considered carefully.

The appropriate patient for student learning at a particular time may not always be available. In fact, the availability of any type of patient is becoming more of a concern in medical schools throughout the world. Even in medical schools that enjoy large patient facilities, the appropriate patient problem frequently is not present or available at a time that would be important for student learning. The available patient, moreover, may present complexities or unrelated problems that can distract or confuse the learner.

Variables in the patient may include uncooperativeness, hostility, difficulties in communication, other disease complications. Although important at some time for learning, these may detract from the immediate value of the patient as a learning experience in certain stages of the student's education. Such variables are uncontrollable and may limit or interfere with educational use.

Patients are available to students only in certain settings, such as hospitals or clinics. These locations may generate significant educational problems, since the student may be seen as only a visitor or even a nuisance by other personnel. Even if ideal, these often are not suitable locations for group discussions, referral to learning resources, self-study, and the repeated study and examination necessary in the early stages of student development. In addition, patients in these settings have to be taken away for diagnostic studies, surgery, therapies, consultations by other health professionals, and often are discharged before the time the student is scheduled for contact with the patient.

Many important types of patient problems that are complex or urgent are not available for student learning because the urgency and seriousness of these problems require immediate and often complex care. Emergency surgery, emergency diagnostic procedures, and a rapid pace of care preclude effective student contact with those kinds of problems, except sometimes as an observer.

Unless the student is relatively skilled and experienced in evaluating patients, the patient may feel as though he is being used as a guinea pig in the student's education. The length of time the student takes, his repeated questions, and the subsequent review by teachers required for student learning may delay patients for inconvenient lengths of time, particularly outpatients. The repeated examination of patients by different students can become fatiguing, particularly for patients that are quite ill or have chronic conditions.

One of the greatest concerns about patients being used educationally is that the inevitable discussions or comments at the side of the patient between students or between students and teacher may inadvertently reveal to the patient information that may not have been discussed with him, such as his prognosis, the significance of some of his complaints, the treatability or untreatability of his disease, or suspected serious conditions. Inept or unskilled questioning of the patient who is anxious, emotionally disturbed, or in other ways upset or hostile about his health situation may be harmful. These unwanted and undesirable effects are more common than most faculty are willing to admit or discover for themselves.

The student himself often is distracted by his neophyte status in front of patients, especially if he has insecure skills in clinical assessment. This embarrassment, combined with concern for harm he might cause the patient, or for a negative reaction to his ministrations, can seriously inhibit the learning that should be occuring with that patient experience.

After the patient has answered repeated questions by different students and has gone through repeated physical examinations and heard repeated discussions, his attitude changes. His history becomes mechanical because it becomes shaped by other's questions; his real worries and concerns are no longer expressed; details are dropped and he becomes passive. The repeated use of patients by students often makes the patient become very "unreal," the opposite of the desired effect.

There has to be a trade-off between the faculty's responsibility for educating students and their responsibility for the comfort of their patients. It is important for students to work with all kinds of patient problems (complex, difficult, urgent, vague, simple, classical, and so forth) and be exposed to these problems in their learning. It also is important that the student observe and experience a variety of symptoms, signs, personalities, and body types, despite some feelings of discomfort, loss of privacy, and delay on the part of the patient. The teachers may have conflicting priorities in their responsibilities to both students and patients. This usually can be handled well by the appropriate preparation of patients for student examinations and preparation of students for their interaction with patients. The teachers constantly must be aware of the fact that their own use of the patient represents a role model for the students. If we expect the student to stress humanity in his work with patients, this must be seen by the student in the teacher's use of patients.

In summary then, the use of the actual patient, although the most relevant and important format for student learning, can have many educational disadvantages. It can be quite harmful to the patient because it can represent a concern only for the student and in many ways may not stress the "humanity" in the application of health care to the patient. It is important that teachers be sensitive to this conflict in priorities and the many other educational drawbacks in the use of patients. Much of this can be resolved by utilizing patient simulations in instances where they offer educational advantages that may be equal to, or even better than, contact with patients. The skills and knowledge gained in work with simulations can then be transferred to real patients by a more skilled and confident student.

Advantages of Using Written Case Histories

The written story of the patient, containing history, physical examination, test results, treatments, and the course of the illness, is a familiar learning format. These written stories can be very brief, containing just the most relevant data; or they can be voluminous, containing the results of comprehensive inquiries or investigations. This ubiquitous problem format is used in clinical pathological conferences, syllabi, textbooks, handouts, lectures, and demonstrations in a wide variety of medical-school courses.

It is probably no coincidence that the advantages and disadvantages of this format are the reverse of those for the real patient in the educational setting. The best problem for a specific group of students at the appropriate complexity or simplicity is available anytime, anywhere. The problem can be studied by the student at any time he wishes and in any place that he desires, at any speed, for any number of times, until the problem has been understood adequately. The student may choose to take on only one aspect of the patient problem. He may choose to make the correct diagnosis, to identify the underlying mechanisms responsible for the symptoms or the disorder, to identify underlying pathology, to order appropriate tests to further elucidate the patient's problem, to interpret tests, or to design a treatment plan, as he wishes. The student can stop at any point, leave the problem, study, then return and apply to the problem what has been learned. He can review the problems as often as necessary. Filed away, the problem is always available for future reference. As the future course of the patient, his response to therapy, his progress, or even autopsy findings usually are known already, the student is able to follow the patient problem to its conclusion or resolution and is able to get feedback as to exactly what the problem was and how it might have been managed best. Since all the elements in the patient's problem are known to the teacher or faculty, criteria for student performance with the problem can be set and appropriate reference materials for student study can be produced, collected, or cited.

Disadvantages of Using Written Case Histories

The educational disadvantages, despite this flexibility in ease of use, are monumental, particularly in light of the clinical reasoning process that the student needs to develop in his work with patient problems. This format is unreal and abstract. There is no challenge to the skills of interview and examination. The patient's appearance, manner, his response to questions, and his findings on examination all are described in words. There is little challenge in making relevant observations about the patient amongst all possible observations in the gestalt of the patient's appearance. All important observations are written down in the abstract, linear format of words.

The student is not challenged to develop an initial concept from initial cues; to generate early hypotheses; or to interview and examine, using an inquiry strategy, in order to rank or verify those hypotheses. All the important patient data usually are provided. In these printed cases, someone else did all the clinical reasoning and made the decision as to what information should be included on the written case history and in what order. The result is a reordering and an abstraction of the data that suited the writer's formulation of the problem but is unfaithful to reality. Over half the challenge offered in a patient problem is denied the student. Elstein et al. (1972) stated an obvious and basic truism about patient problems as they present to the physician, saying, "all the important information needed to solve problems is typically unavailable." In written case histories, it is made available.

The skill of the physician is to obtain the information needed through his skills in clinical reasoning. With this type of format the student has little freedom in working with the problem, outside of interpreting and analyzing the data presented and hypothesizing the possible underlying pathophysiology or disease process. The challenge to his clinical reasoning can be improved if the facts or data in the case are presented in a serial fashion and the student has an opportunity at each stage to decide what he would do next before reading the next section (this is the so-called sequential management problem). Nevertheless, even though he decides on the tests he might order or the treatments he might employ, he can never see the consequences of his own decisions because the next segment reveals what the clinician responsible for the problem did. As conventionally used, this format has limited usefulness and provides low motivation to students.

Problem Simulations

One solution to this dilemma in problem formats would be to have available on demand, at any time and in any location, patients who present specified problems. Ideally, they would be patients in whom all the relevant data and facts about their clinical picture were known, as well as their future course or outcomes. These patients would not require medical attention and could tolerate repeated student examination and discussion. At the same time, they would be able to challenge the student's clinical reasoning, clinical skills, and interpersonal skills. They would present specific medical, social, and emotional problems and would not vary from student to student. They would present urgent and complex problems to which the student could apply his skills fully without competing for urgent health-care needs on the part of the patient, so that even with an urgent problem the student could take his time or repeat his approaches until his skills were secure.

Another solution would incorporate the advantages of the written case history by being portable and easily useable and reuseable. This would be a printed version of the patient that would challenge all the aspects of the student's clinical reasoning skills. This format should allow him to follow the consequences of his decisions or actions with the patient and should also, by the use of audiovisual media, allow him to make observations about the patient's appearances and the results of such tests as X rays or specimens.

If these solutions were possible, the advantages of the real patient and the printed case history could be realized without their disadvantages, and each would complement the other educationally. They would help to develop both the student's clinical reasoning skills and self-directed study skills. The patient would be available for the development of the psychomotor aspects of his clinical and interpersonal skills and the printed format would be available for use anywhere at any time.

Living Patients

The first goal, that of developing the student's clinical reasoning skills, is accomplished by the use of simulated patients (Barrows, 1971). Simulated patients are normal people who are specially trained, by a specific yet not complex method similar to "method acting," to simulate an actual patient in every detail. This training allows them to reproduce a patient's problem as if it were their own, so that they are able to appear, move, and respond to any question as the patient would. They present the same emotional or attitudinal picture as the actual patient. In the training of the simulated patient, care is taken not to sophisticate them with any medical information about the illness or patient they are portraying, beyond what a lay person would normally learn. They learn to take on the patient's problem as a life role. In this way, they behave as real patients without knowledge that would bias their performances or make them seem artificial. In addition, simulated patients can be taught to simulate a surprising variety of physical findings, such as coma, seizures, lid lag, tremors, absent or abnormal breath sounds, muscle spasms, weakness, altered reflexes, abdominal tenderness, thyroid bruit, blindness, and the like. This range enlarges as creative teachers work more and more with this variety of simulation.

In addition, there are many patients who describe symptoms on interview that require the student to perform a careful physical examination, even though there are ultimately no physical findings. This could occur in anginal pain, back pain, abdominal pain, vertigo, episodic weakness, complaints of fatigue, diarrhea, and the like. There are varied and effective simulations in almost every specialty or area of medicine, with the exception perhaps of neonatology. Children have been simulated effectively down to the age of nine. Psychiatric simulations also have proved to be feasible and very effective.

Any kind of patient problem can be simulated: straightforward, classic cases; confusing, bizarre problems; vague, difficult-to-understand problems;

common problems; or rare problems. The important point is that all simulations are based on actual cases. The use of actual patients as training models allows the clinician who cared for the actual case to assist in the simulation and to be certain that the final product is an authentic replica of the real patient. Students working with such a simulation can be assured that such a problem really existed and that they are working with a problem that does occur in medical practice. The course of the actual patient is known. This information, together with all the tests and diagnostic procedures that were done on the real patient, can be used to create resources for extending the teaching or evaluation of clinical skills with the simulated patient problem.

It has been well established on many occasions that simulated patients cannot be differentiated from actual patients by even experienced clinicians (Burri et al., 1976). Over the last 15 years, this teaching tool has grown in use, for both teaching and evaluation at undergraduate, postgraduate, and continuing medical educational levels. The teacher has an unvarying patient problem that can be scheduled for the student learning at any time and in any location.

One of the most potent advantages of the simulated patient over real patients is the unbiased feedback they can provide to the student about their personal reactions to his professional approach and manner during the encounter. Simulated patients can be given instructions on how to provide this feedback, from the patient's point of view, in a constructive manner. Patients, because they are in the patient role and dependent upon the health-care system, can never do this in such an unbiased manner. Feedback directly from the simulated patient appears to be more accurate than third-party observation of the interaction between the student and the patient. Experience over a number of years has shown repeatedly that considerable interpersonal communication can occur between physician and patient that is not apparent to even the most sensitive observer watching through a one-way glass or viewing a videotape. This aspect of simulated patients has proved to be universally appealing to students because they can have their skills and manner evaluated at no risk.

The training of simulated patients is rather easy, once the technique has been seen and tried by the teacher. It requires far less time and effort than is commonly supposed.

Paper Patients

A variety of formats have been designed so that the written case history can provide a more realistic challenge to the student's reasoning skills. This also can be called a simulation, since the attempt is to represent more realistically the clinical situation for the student. Maatch (1974) has discriminated among simulations in medicine by their "fidelity" to the patient's setting. With this schema, patients would be at the top and simulated patients immediately below. The case history would be at the bottom. Many new formats for the written problem have been designed, in an attempt to raise the fidelity of the printed format. Initial efforts in this area were stimulated by the need for more effective or valid evaluation of students' clinical reasoning or problem-solving skills. (Hubbard et al., 1965; Williamson, 1965; McGuire & Babbott, 1967), and by a need to evaluate students' skills for teaching and research purposes (Rimoldi, 1972; de Dombal et al., 1972; Helfer & Slater, 1971). These printed, easily reproduced, relatively inexpensive, portable formats can be used by single students, groups, or large classes, in a variety of settings. Although they originally were designed in many instances to evaluate students, they are particularly ideal for individualized, self-paced, self-directed study and for the development of clinical reasoning skills. They can be used for student evaluation by the student himself or by the teacher, either for individual student's evaluation or evaluation of the teaching program. When these formats are used for learning, the student may leave them at any stage to pursue further discussion or study and then return to them for application of the necessary acquired information and skills.

Some of the more commonly used of these formats are the PMP or "patient management problems," the SMP or "sequential management problems," and, more recently, the P4 or "*portable patient problem pack*." These are prototypic models; many variations of each exist. For example, both Rimoldi (1972), de Dombal et al. (1972), and Helfer & Slater (1971) have utilized a card fromat for measuring the problem-solving process. These units are quite similar to the P4. The "problem box" used at McMaster University would now be called a sequential management problem (Barrows & Mitchell, 1975). A variety of study materials often were included in the box.

The PMP. This is one of the most common formats. It presents an initial picture of the patient to the student and then offers him a series of options from which he chooses his subsequent inquiry (history, physical examination items, tests, or treatments). These options are offered in categories of actions following the patient exposition. After the student chooses one of the options, the results of that choice are revealed either through rub-out or latent-image techniques. The student is then referred to another section in the PMP where more information about the patient is revealed and he is confronted again with new choices to make as the patient problem unfolds. The student is able to see the consequences of his own decision. He can follow the problem until it has either been successfully or unsuccessfully managed. During the course of his work with the problem, the student can order diagnostic tests, procedures, and treatment plans, and see how the patient has fared as a consequence of these interventions. Complications can arise that the student has to manage as they occur. Branching in this format can become very complex but, nevertheless, it is easily administered and scored for large groups of students. It has the disadvantage of cueing the student, in that a choice of several alternative actions is made available to him at each section that may suggest approaches he may not have thought of by himself. There is an additional artificiality in that the student has to choose one of the responses offered before he can move to the next section of the problem. The available options may not represent any of the actions he would like to perform with the actual patient at that time.

The SMP. The sequential management problem also presents the student with an initial picture of the patient and then may offer the student a series of choices from options that have been listed as in the PMP. In some SMP formats, however, he may be free to write down his assessment and actions on a blank page. In the SMP, once the student has made his choice or committed himself, he then turns to the next segment of the patient's course, regardless of the action he chose. In this new segment, he is told what actions were taken in the actual case, what the results were, and what the physician's thinking was at that time. Then more of the patient problem is unfolded for new actions or decisions to be made. In both these formats, many aspects of the clinical reasoning process are challenged, such as cue perception, developing an initial concept, generating hypotheses, and choosing appropriate actions within certain constraints. The advantage to the SMP format is that the student is not forced to follow a blind alley should he make incorrect decisions as to what he would do next or how he would handle the case. By comparing what he did with what actually occurred, he can evaluate at each segment the wisdom of his choice, or his thinking. In the SMP, the student can be carried through a whole sequence of experiences with a problem while gaining feedback at each step; however, he has the disadvantage of a "linear" program in which he is not able to express and gain feedback from the patient for his own clinical reasoning since he is forced to follow someone else's course. By contrast, the PMP allows the student to follow the consequences of his own decisions without any feedback or guidance during the course of the problem. Each has specific educational advantages over the other, depending upon the nature of the educational goals of the student or teacher.

The P4. More recently, the authors have produced the P4 as a card format designed to overcome some of the problems inherent in both the SMP and the PMP (Barrows & Tamblyn, 1977). This format allows the student to take any action possible with the real patient, in any sequence he feels appropriate. As in the real clinical situation, the student is able to see the result of each action before deciding on the next and is challenged to evaluate and manage the patient's problem appropriately. He is as free to make mistakes, perform unnecessary tests, or order incorrect treatments as he is to manage the problem effectively.

The P4 units consist of a deck of several hundred cards in a variety of colors, including photograph cards of the same size. The colors categorize the type of action that can be taken with the patient. The white cards are all the possible questions that might be asked on history; blue cards are all the actions that might be taken on physical examination; orange cards are all the laboratory tests that might be requested; green cards are all the consultants and other sources of information that the clinician might want to use in his evaluation; pink cards are all the treatments or interventions he might like to utilize. The assembled titles of these several hundred cards represent all the possible or conceivable actions the student might want to take with any patient problem, not just those that may be relevant to the case at hand. Only a small percentage of the cards are necessary in working effectively with the patient problem presented in a specific deck, minimizing cueing.

Below the title of each card is a series of questions designed to stimulate the student's clinical reasoning process. They ask him how he has put the problem together at this point (formulation), what his hypotheses are, and what actions he wants to take next (ask a question, examine, order a test, or stop and study: inquiry strategy).

The backs of the cards give the student the patient's or others' responses to the action indicated by the front title: answers to his questions (white cards), findings on physical examination (blue cards), results of investigations (orange cards), opinion of consultants (green cards), and the results of the interventions or treatments (pink cards). The student may be referred to appropriate photograph cards of X rays, patient appearance, views of the fundi, displays of isotope scans, or other laboratory tests, for him to interpret. The interpretation of these investigations is printed upside down on the back of the card to prevent the student from accidentally reading it until he has tried to interpret the studies himself.

The first card the student reads is the "situation card," which initiates his work with the patient problem. This card states how the patient problem presents itself and in what setting. On the basis of this card, he then has to determine what his actions will be in evaluating and treating the patient problem. There is also a closure card, which the student draws when he feels he has finished his encounter with the patient and does not care to take any more actions. It is easy to see how the P4 is designed to facilitate the clinical reasoning process described previously.

There is a separate series of cards, the P3 or "patient progress pack." These cards are in the format of a sequential management problem, to allow the student to manage the patient's problem over time, once he has evaluated it in the P4 format.

The P4 is associated with a variety of evaluation tools that the student or the teacher may use. Some show the sequence of P4 cards chosen by a variety of experts in various fields of medicine and nursing, for the student to compare with his own. He has formulas similar to the ones available in the PMP's to evaluate his proficiency, economy of actions, and other factors in his clinical reasoning process. This unit can be utilized by individual students, pairs of students, groups of students, or classes in a variety of settings. More details of this format will be given in Chapter 7.

Computer Formats. A variety of computer formats have also been developed to present problems to students (Harless et al., 1971; Friedman et al., 1973, 1977; Dickinson et al., 1973). Many of these computer formats can challenge the student's clinical reasoning in all of its segments by displaying the evolving information about the patient on a video screen or by typewriter. The student can ask questions, request items of physical examination, and order tests, and the results of his actions are displayed for him to read. There is no cueing with this format and the student is free to take any action he wants. More important, the computer can be programmed to produce changes in the patient's picture over time, putting even more realism into the problem and challenging the student's patient-care skills, particularly with acute or urgent problems.

The "Mac" series developed at McMaster University requires the student to work with changing, interlocking physiological parameters, as in respiratory disorders, renal diseases, and drug overdose. The effect of any treatment intervention on other physiological functions or parameters is displayed (Dickinson et al., 1973). There are distinct advantages offered by the computer in its ability to handle concurrently a number of simultaneous temporal events and their interrelationships, and to produce spontaneous changes in the patient status over time. The disadvantage of computers relates to the expense involved in their operation, the often complex and difficult method of interaction with a computer, and the fact that they are fixed in one location. These disadvantages are being overcome, however, by the use of newer technologies.

The value of all these formats can be enhanced by the integration of audiovisual media. Pictures or videotapes of the patient can challenge the student's observation skills, as can images of fundi, skin lesions, responses of the patient to examination procedures, and the like. Images of X rays, scans, histological specimens, electrocardiograms, and electroencephalograms, can be reproduced to challenge the student's skills in the interpretation of tests.

There is a wide variety of models made of plastic and other materials that simulate physical findings in the abdomen, breasts, pelvis, and back. There are heads with replaceable retinal images that can be viewed by an ophthalmoscope. Heart sounds, bowel sounds, and chest sounds can be recorded on audiotape and listened to through a stethoscope arrangement. All of these can be used to extend the simulation of a patient's problem for student learning and evaluation.

Many of these simulations can be integrated around a single patient problem, combining their advantages. In all of these simulated formats, it is only the simulated patient that, short of actual patients, can challenge the student's interpersonal skills and psychomotor skills of interview and examination of a patient. Educational advantages can be achieved by combining students' interactions with the simulated patient with another format such as the PMP, P4, or computer. This allows the student to take the data base and problem formulation he obtains from his examination and interview of a simulated patient and request tests or diagnostic investigations, begin treatment, and follow the patient over time. Not one of these simulated patients, however, can be thought of as a substitute for the real patient. The educational advantages of simulation formats allow the student to learn and to develop reasoning and examination skills by repeated work with simulations until a certain mastery is achieved. The skills that he gains from simulations can be transferred to work with real patients for more advanced experiences and learning. His experiences with simulation will allow him to work with real patients without concern or distractions because of insecure techniques or skills. The real patient usually is not discomforted by student examinations if the student is relatively skilled and seems capable of contributing to his care. The more skillful student is not seen as someone who is using him as a "guinea pig" for learning.

These formats of simulation are abstracted from the real world to allow the student to develop skills at no risk. They represent educationally sound ways of transferring the student to his real world task. This is the role of simulation in many areas of learning outside of medicine. The complex and expensive simulations of airline cockpits, locomotive cockpits, and spacecraft and navigational trainers are used for the same purpose. The student learns progressively complex skills in a realistic situation, but at no risk. These are skills that he will be able to transfer effectively to the real task situation because they were learned in a setting that is faithful to many aspects of the real world. These simulations, as in medical simulations, allow for accurate, recurrent and personalized evaluation. It is an educational truism that the more real the learning environment, compared to the ultimate task environment, the more effective will be the transfer of skills to real tasks (Jason et al., 1971).

A last and most important aspect of these simulations as a method of teaching in undergraduate education is their ability to stress the "humanity" of patient care. No matter what the educational goals of the student or the faculty may be, the student has to be able to take care of the concerns and problems presented by the whole patient. If the student undertakes a problem-based learning unit, a simulated patient, or a P4 format in order to gain an understanding in neuroanatomy, he still has to deal with the patient's symptoms, life situation, and concerns, in his evaluation of the problem. The student has to develop interpersonal skills. Using patient simulations as a focus for teaching in undergraduate education always reinforces the need for being sensitive to the entire patient in both learning and in practice.

CHAPTER 5

Facilitating Problem-Based Learning and the Development of Clinical Reasoning Skills for the Teacher and Student

The facilitation of both clinical reasoning and self-directed study requires an awareness of the process of clinical reasoning and an appropriate patient problem. Each of these requirements has been discussed in the previous chapters. Although teachers and students have a wide variety of options available within the problem-based teaching–learning process, the basic sequence for problem-based learning can be described as follows.

1. Identification of the objectives of the session
2. Interaction with the patient problem
3. Identification of self-study questions raised by work with the problem
4. Self-directed study
5. Application of acquired information back to the problem
6. Review and synthesis of what has been learned
7. Evaluation

This process will be considered in this chapter and the next.

Using the Simulated Patient to Illustrate the Process

The problem-based learning setting that will be described here as an initial example is that of a small group of four to five students, a teacher, and a simulated patient. This particular situation is chosen because it allows

71

the basic techniques involved in facilitating proglem-based learning to be seen most clearly, and because it can be used with students at all levels. The approach described in this setting can be adapted to the use of a variety of other patient simulations, such as case histories, P4s, PMPs, and SMPs. This approach also can be adapted to different numbers of students, can be used in a classroom setting, and can even be employed by students in their own self-directed study program or by a group of students who have gained the skills necessary to work on their own without a teacher.

Defining Educational Objectives

Before students begin problem-based learning with a simulated patient, a few basic questions need to be answered. Is the problem being studied in order to learn

1. Clinical skills?
2. Interpersonal skills?
3. Diagnosis, differential diagnosis, or problem formulation and treatment?
4. Basic mechanisms, pathophysiological or psychological?
5. Concepts or information from science areas related to the problem (anatomy, physiology, epidemiology, pathology)?

Of course, the objectives could include one or more of those as stated above, or others. It is important that objectives be identified to ensure that the course followed by the group in their work with the problem accomplishes them. Objectives can be those stated for the curriculum or course in which the students are presently studying or objectives specified by the teacher in a teacher-centered approach. In a student-centered approach, the individual student's personal objectives, the stated course objectives, and the knowledge acquired from work with prior problems can be used to formulate objectives. Particular problems may be selected because they involve the student in particular areas of science or clinical medicine. The identification of objectives is important as any patient problem could lead to study or research to a wide variety of areas presenting a formidable and even endless task in learning. Objectives provide a focus. The student group also might become preoccupied with activities that are not appropriate to their learning at the particular time. A common example is a tendency for students, even early in the curriculum, to become preoccupied with the challenge of making a clinical diagnosis when the identification of basic mechanisms and the acquisition of information from the basic sciences are the appropriate objectives. In the student's work with the problem, the hypotheses created, the problem formulations developed, and the study areas identified would vary depending upon these stated objectives. Although the establishment of objectives may sound like an involved process, it becomes automatic with practice.

Defining the Learning Atmosphere

The teacher must help the students understand that there are no right or wrong answers with this kind of learning. No one in the group is to be censured, criticized, or marked down for making naive or "dumb" statements. There should be no attempt on the part of students or teachers to cover up areas of ignorance. If there is something that a student does not know or is unsure of, he should say so readily. It is only in this climate that learning appropriate for the individual student can occur. Physicians are not infallible or all-knowing, and many of the medical principles and concepts on which practice is based are often vague, poorly established, or looked upon differently by different experts. Learning can occur only when ignorance or lack of knowledge is freely admitted. Also, the freedom required to aggressively create a variety of possible hypotheses to explain the problem is severely inhibited if the student is afraid to show ignorance or will not speak unless he has all the facts. This climate is best established by the teacher admitting his own ignorance in the explorations that ensue, without resorting to the academic defenses for ignorance usually used in front of students, such as, "why don't you look that up," or "let's bring that up at another time." Openly admitting you don't know allows for learning to occur.

Cooperation

The group must agree on sharing the responsibilities for the group's success in working with a problem. This requires that they all actively work towards evaluating the problem, identifying self-directed issues, learning information that is applicable to the problem and that will be helpful to the rest of the group, and evaluating the group's and their own efforts in these endeavors. The sharing of mutual support and criticism given openly and honestly is crucial to the success of problem-based learning. As each student becomes aware of other students' backgrounds and career aspirations, as well as their individual learning habits or styles, he can complement and reinforce the others in the group process. Each must feel responsible, along with the teacher, if the group process bogs down or becomes nonproductive. This responsibility of each member of the group helps the students develop their personal ability to both evaluate their own abilities and work constructively with others.

The Use of the Simulated Patient

Ground rules for the educational use of the simulated patient also need to be established. The students must realize that the simulation is based upon a real patient and is faithful to the picture that the patient presented. Since it is a simulated patient, there is no need for the students to be concerned about making mistakes or about asking questions or performing examinations that might upset the patient. They need to understand that the interaction with the simulated patient can be interrupted for discussion by the group. During these "time outs" for group discussion, the simulated patient will remain in role but will behave as if the group is not there and when "time in" is declared will continue on as if no interruption had occurred. This allows discussion to occur between the students and teacher to analyze and critique each others' reasoning and identify educational needs at frequent intervals in the course of their work with the problem.

The simulated patient provides the educational advantages of challenging the student's interpersonal, interviewing, and examination skills. It requires the students to be concerned for the whole person, as well as the problem under study; to care about someone who must be understood and made comfortable during the encounter. The students have to be sensitive to the patient's concerns and his responses to their ministrations, and must evaluate and deal with the patient's total problem, medical and psychosocial. As a last ground rule, therefore, the students must behave during "time in" as they would in the presence of a real patient, so that interpersonal skills and sensitivities can be studied and critiqued by the group.

Usually, the teacher will tell the students the setting in which they are confronting the simulated patient; that is, in the emergency room, clinic, hospital ward, or whatever. In addition, the teacher may, depending upon the problem and the educational goals involved, provide other background information that normally might be available with such a patient. One student, who has agreed to start the interaction with the patient, opens the interview while the rest of the students watch. The teacher must always keep the model discussed in Chapter 3 (Figures 3-1 through 3-4) in his mind as he watches the student interview the patient. The point at which the teacher decides on a "time out" to stop the interview with the patient depends upon what he sees occurring and where he feels such a break for discussion by the group might bring to light salient points or insights, or identify problems in the clinical reasoning process. When these discussions occur, the teacher has to resist telling the students what he thinks is wrong or lecturing them on the appropriate questions, techniques, concepts, or information needed at that particular time. Instead, the teacher must serve as a guide, a Socrates, a "tutor," and, through skillful questions and challenges, allow the students to critique their own approaches and develop insights about the adequacy of their thinking or reasoning. This is not to say that the teacher avoids making occasional observations or avoids providing facts at crucial points to facilitate the progress of the group, but he always must be certain that the burden of learning in this format is on the students. More detail concerning this skill will be considered again in this chapter; it represents the most important teaching skills for faculty involved in problem-based learning.

Facilitating Discussion Using the Reasoning Process

After the first student has asked a number of questions of the patient, the teacher may decide to stop for a "time out" discussion or may decide that enough interaction has gone on and that a discussion of the student's cognitive processes at this point could help the group to look at the initial stages of the clinical reasoning process. During this time out, the interviewing student can review aloud what information he acquired from the patient. Then the teacher can ask the other students in the group if they agree with the first student's summary of the information. Had they noted any additional information and would they summarize the patient's situation any differently? The teacher can concentrate here on the richness and accuracy of the *initial cues* perceived by the students. He can determine if the students have looked at all the information that might be available from the setting, the patient's appearance, his movements, his speech, and his manners, as well as his words. The teacher can encourage the students to be consciously aware of all the types and sources of information that are initially available to them. The teacher also can see if there is any unconscious bias in the interpretations made of these initial cues. Have the students "stereotyped" the patient or made any premature judgments or interpretations of what the patient may have said or intended?

Next, the teacher can ask the interviewing student to sum up his *initial concept* of the patient's problem as he sees it at this time and see if this fits with the other students' concepts. In this summary, the teacher can see if all the pertinent positive or negative information obtained to this point has been concisely assembled, is without sophistication unwarranted by the available data, and is free of interpreter bias.

The group then can be asked to review what ideas they might have to explain the problem they have summarized to this point: to make *hypotheses*. In the early years of medical school, students may have only a most limited idea of possible diagnoses, so they often tend to opt for psychological or psychiatric causes for almost any complaint since they usually feel their medical knowledge or experience is too limited. When the teacher collects the ideas from four or five students, however, utilizing their combined back-ground experiences, a wider range of possibilities usually can be brought forth as hypotheses.

At this point, the teacher can stimulate creativity or divergent thinking by asking the group to brainstorm possible hypotheses. Despite protestations by the students that they do not have enough knowledge to do this, the teacher can unlock vast treasures of ideas that come from students' past experiences with medicine in their prior schooling, from relatives, from medical friends, from their readings, from television, and a wide variety of other sources. It is at this point that the students must be reminded that there should be no concern for foolish or dumb statements and that it is only with a rich and wide range of possibilities that you can select the most prob-able or feasible hypotheses to pursue. Once a variety of hypotheses have been decided upon (at least more than two), the students can be asked how these hypotheses should be ranked in their importance. With skillfully monitored discussion by the teacher, even first-year students usually will come up with concerns about probability, life-threatening potential, and treatability. Once the pool of hypotheses has been decided upon, the teacher can ask the stu-dents how the subsequent inquiry of the patient can be best designed to help rule in or rule out these hypotheses. What questions should be asked, in what order, and what effect will possible answers to these questions have on rea-soning? The teacher can identify here the need to develop skills in vertical thinking or deductive reasoning.

Hypotheses Should Match the Educational Goals

It may be assumed incorrectly at this point that the generation of hypotheses in this facilitation of clinical reasoning refers to diagnostic or clinical hypotheses and that problem-based learning around patient problems inevitably leads to clinical learning and not to effective basic science learning. The hypotheses developed depend on the educational objectives. If learning around a patient problem is being used to accomplish basic science objectives, then the hypotheses developed by the students in response to the patient data elicited should be those of altered form or functions at a level appro-priate to the stated objective. For example, the hypotheses can concern possi-ble anatomical (organ, tissue), physiological, biochemical, or molecular events or alterations that may be responsible for the problem(s) identified at that point. They also could concern the possible psychological, sociological, or epidemiological mechanisms responsible for the problem. If clinical learning, diagnostic evaluation, and therapy are objectives, then the hypotheses can refer to possible pathological processes, etiologies, disease states, or organ derangements, as appropriate.

Continuing the Process

During the time that discussion goes on between student and teacher about students' clinical reasoning, the simulated patient maintains the appearance of the actual patient but acts as if unaware of any of the comments by the group or of the passage of time. In the real clinical situation, the cognitive actions under discussion may have gone on in the clinician's mind within a matter of seconds. The "time out" allows this activity to be dissected for its full educational value. When "time in" occurs, another student might be given the challenge to continue with the inquiry using as a guide the *formulation* and *hypotheses* developed by the group. During the discussions in "time out," the students may be given the further challenge of not only looking at the active student's inquiry but also at his interpersonal skills in working with the patient.

After sufficient inquiry has occurred, or a particularly important point has surfaced, the next student can be asked to take a "time out." The "time out" and "time in" convention must be adhered to so that the student always realizes that such discussions should not happen in front of real patients. Once the students are experienced in this procedure of discussion with time outs, they usually begin calling for them on their own initiative. Either the student who is interviewing the patient feels that an appropriate time out should be taken, or the students observing the interaction feel that it is time for the discussion. It is important for the students to develop skills in the facilitation of clinical reasoning so that they can apply it to their own individual work with problems. At each new time out, the discussion can consider the new data obtained from the simulated patient, its reliability, and its effect on the evolving problem formulation and the hypotheses generated. Eventually, enough data will be accumulated so that the initial concept can be enlarged into an evolving *problem formulation.* A student can be asked to present his formulation of the patient's problem, as he sees it, for subsequent discussion by the group.

The teacher should not regiment the discussion by directly saying such things as "What is the problem formulation?" Instead, he should ask, "What new information do we have now that could be helpful? How does this affect the initial statement we made about the patient's problem? Should it be changed? What effect does this new information have on the few ideas we had about the actual cause of the problem? Can we eliminate some? Do we need to modify any? Are there new ones to be considered?" and so forth. All this time, the teacher is looking at the quality of the student's processes and such possible pathologies as those described in Chapter 2 that may need to be identified, discussed, and modified. As this process is really an analysis of a common-sense lifetime skill, the student, if properly guided, eventually will make all the observations and suggestions that the teacher would have made. The group constantly should look for observations that may have been overlooked, possible biassed in the interpretation of these observations, translation errors, and poorly formed formulations. The *problem formulation* should encompass all the significant positive and negative data from the patient situation at any given point in the process. The daily hypotheses usually should be broad, numerous, and clearly stated. All the data obtained must be weighed against both the growing formulation and the hypotheses. In addition, the group should look at how effective each interviewer is in designing an inquiry that is aimed at eliminating or ranking these hypotheses, as well as his interpersonal skill in facilitating communication and in making the patient comfortable. It's amazing how clearly the student's thinking is exposed and how easily errors or problems in his approach to a patient problem can be seen in this simulation–discussion format. The teacher can see things that can never be seen in any other setting. For example, even though the formulations and hypotheses have been agreed upon by the students, the subsequent inquiry of the patient may not be guided by these hypotheses. Instead, the students may automatically ask questions they have learned to ask in the past, without applying any discipline in deductive reasoning.

Enlarging the Inquiry Strategy

At some point, the students will have to decide that they have obtained from the interview all the information they need to aid their reasoning at that point and that they now need to turn to other sources of information, such as the physical examination or certain laboratory or diagnostic tests, to continue their evaluation and management of the problem. The students may not realize this themselves, but it will become clear to the teacher that they are not going to be able to refine their hypotheses or develop their formulations any further by continuing the interview. Comments such as "Where are we going?" or "Do you think we are making any progress?" can be made to the students. Hopefully, several students will have sensed the fact that they seem to be going in circles and are making no new progress, and will express their concern that no new information seems to be forthcoming. The question then can be raised as to when the clinician should move on to such other sources of information as the physical examination and how should this decision be made. When the students decide to examine the patient — a tense and difficult step for students with no patient experience — they can be asked about what they will look for in the physical examination to further process their hypotheses or to sharpen their problem formulation. This type of question makes it clear that the physical examination is not a technical ritual to be imposed on the patient, but, like the history, is another method of data acquisition to be used relevant to hypotheses about the patient. In time, with other problems, this direct search for data relevant to hypotheses about the patient can be brought out and contrasted to the use of questions and examinations as a scanning or screening technique to seek other cues about possibly unrelated or unsuspected problems. The most important skills the students need, however, are to be able to decide upon an effective inquiry strategy that derives the data necessary to rank, refine, and verify hypotheses. The particular choice of question, item on physical examinations, or test to be done, and the sequence should depend on the data needed to analyze the hypotheses.

Physical Examination Skills

The introduction of beginning students to the physical examination in this simulated-patient/small-group format can be stimulating and productive. The teacher can assure the students that the simulated patient does not object to examination and that no one has any expectations that they should know how to do a proper examination. The challenge is for the students to be aware of their hypotheses, to apply what they already know about medicine to the body, and to figure out what they would like to examine and how. A selection of diagnostic tools can be available, but only minimal guidance in their use is needed. It is surprising how sophisticated students can be in selecting the appropriate actions in examination. They invariably become motivated to learn the appropriate examination techniques, during subsequent self-study time, from the many resources that are available. The important fact is that they see the physical examination in the same light as their interview; an extension of their cognitive reasoning processes. They develop the ability to think on their feet while they work with the patient problem, and do not just mechanically examine the patient without an idea of what needs to be sought and how. The student soon learns that if he isn't looking for something he probably won't find it. With more sophisticated or advanced students, you can ask not only what they expect to look for in the examination of the patient but also what they expect to find in their examinations of the patient, based on the information they have obtained so far.

Hopefully the students eventually will feel free to move back and forth between the history and physical, as appropriate, to sort out the hypotheses that are in their minds. They should discover that one physical finding may save minutes of nonproductive interview, because there are many symptoms that are hard to understand or characterize on interview alone.

Summing Up the Simulated-Patient Experience

During the entire time that the students are working with the problem presented by the simulated patient, the teacher and students should strive for the following.

1. Accuracy and thoroughness of perceptions and observations
2. Proper interpretation, synthesis, and translation of the information perceived or observed
3. Elimination of possible unconscious biases produced by incorrect or poorly fitting medical labels being applied to the information obtained or the problem formulations developed
4. Elimination of possible biases in thinking caused by stereotyping the patient or by preconceptions about the type of problem the patient may have from the situation he presents (as, for example, the "neurotic housewife" or the "irresponsible teenager")
5. Accuracy in the hypotheses developed, relevant to educational goals. If the goals were to develop an understanding of the basic mechanisms, then the hypotheses should reflect concepts of disordered anatomy, physiology, biochemistry, psychological mechanisms, and the like. If the goals were those of clinical evaluation and management, they should relate to disorders, diseases, syndromes, and organ systems, as well as to disordered form and function
6. Conciseness and accuracy in the problem formulation as a continuous summary of all the relevant positive and negative information obtained from the patient
7. Data search or inquiry strategy that is relevant to the hypotheses being considered, eliminating some while verifying or ranking others
8. Discipline in applying the information obtained on inquiry against the hypotheses. The significance of the data in weakening or strengthening hypotheses should be recognized and the hypotheses modified accordingly
9. Appropriate use of scanning techniques, when a blind alley is reached in reasoning with the patient problem, in searching for new cues or other possibilities
10. Appropriate use of interview and examination techniques to obtain valid and reliable data
11. Appropriate use of interpersonal skills to establish communication with and comfort for the patient
12. Consideration of the whole patient as a person, including his multiple problems, both medical and psychosocial

13. Identification of the group's deficiencies in knowledge or skills as areas of further study.

This list is not at all complete, nor can all these things be considered at any one particular time or with every problem. The list indicates areas that can be focused on to develop and refine the students' thinking. Although the teacher can carry the burden of these concerns in early work with the students, the students themselves should begin to take on more and more responsibility for evaluating and critiquing their own approaches and those of their peers. The eventual goal, as stated previously, is that the individual student can continue to critique and develop his own skills.

Concern for the Whole Patient

As the evaluation of the patient's problem continues, it is necessary to be sure that all the patient's concerns are met in the encounter. It is important for students at all levels of learning to be involved in this essential part of the encounter, even if their main learning goals are in basic science. Concern for the whole patient, his needs, his rights, and his expectations, must become automatic from the outset. If the goals of the encounter include treatment or management of the patient's problem, the students should entertain hypotheses concerning the various treatment or management plans that could be appropriate. After they have evaluated the patient problem, they should make decisions in the same manner as they did with their hypotheses related to evaluation. This may require more inquiry from the patient concerning his ability or willingness to follow the plan, conflicts with other medications, ability to leave job and come to the hospital, and the like. The effects of proposed hospitalization or involved diagnostic investigations need to be reviewed. Eventually, decisions have to be made as to what management plan will be undertaken. The patient should be informed appropriately of the conclusions of the evaluation. The treatment plan needs to be considered if the group has clinical goals. The skills necessary to ensure compliance by educating the patient can be developed with the simulated patient.

Decision Making

As this work with a simulated patient progresses, the point at which closure occurs needs to be considered. Eventually, a decision needs to be made that either all the information that is appropriate to evaluate the problem has been obtained or that no more information is available at this time and further evaluation is going to depend upon laboratory investigations, consultations, or response to treatment on subsequent re-evaluation. In the simulated patient setting, the educational goals determine this end point. For example, if the goals were to elucidate underlying mechanisms to the problem (altered anatomy, physiology, or biology), then closure would occur when the group felt that they had gotten as far as they could go, considering the data available or their own knowledge base. The educational goals also could be in other nonclinical areas, such as understanding underlying epidemiology, pathology, or health-care delivery concepts. If, however, the students have taken on the problem for clinical goals of evaluation and management, then, as in the actual clinical situation, closure will occur when this has been decided upon. If the patient situation is found to be urgent or life threatening, closure will represent the point at which intervention for crucial investigations or treatments should occur and where unnecessary evaluation should be curtailed. The simulation of emergency problems forces the student to identify inquiry actions that have the highest information yields and interventions that aim at the highest payoff in terms of life or well being. At closure, self-directed learning issues and evaluation of the exercise are considered.

None of these educational goals need to be influenced by the student's level in the curriculum. Basic science learning goals may be valuable for clinical or postgraduate students; clinical goals may be valuable for learning in the early years, depending upon the educational goals developed by the group.

Self-Directed Learning

Although the skills of self-directed learning have been separated here from the development of clinical reasoning skills, it should be apparent that in this mode of learning the students constantly will face areas where knowledge is lacking. Examples include the knowledge necessary to think of other possible hypotheses, to interpret symptoms or complaints, to evaluate the data against the hypotheses, and to determine how to ask certain questions that will test hypotheses. As these educational problems appear, the choice of which of several learning options to use will depend upon the group's goals and the time available.

Students should write down the questions that have been raised during the problem inquiry. As necessary in the real clinical situation, the student should be encouraged to move on with the problem as far as possible, despite a lack of specific information, and see how far his own reasoning and knowledge base will take him. This is consistent with the skills the clinician must have, since he always will be faced with novel and unusual problems. Occasionally, the teacher may offer some facts or suggestions to facilitate students' progress with the problem. This should be done judiciously and usually at the specific request of the students, keeping them responsible for their learning. A brief recourse to nearby textbooks or dictionary may be helpful.

Reasoning is no longer possible, however, when the group has run out of facts with which to put the problem together. If it is clear that too many questions have been raised about the patient problem or that further work with the problem is impossible, the decision should be made for the group to stop for a period of appropriate self-directed study and then return to the problem. It is important to stop before students become frustrated by their inability to understand the problem and at a point at which the desire to know or the frustration of limited knowledge provides a strong stimulus for productive study. The students can agree to continue with the problem at a later time when the new information can be applied. The concept of this student-centered/self-directed study will be picked up later in this chapter.

The Teacher as Facilitator

A closer look at the teacher's role in this type of learning can be made at this point, although it will be dealt with in more detail at the end of the chapter. The learning required of the student is active, not passive. The student does not listen, observe, write, and memorize; instead, he is asked to perform, think, get involved, commit himself, and learn by trial and error. He is asked to learn both cognitive reasoning skills and the psycho-motor skills of interview and examination, and to identify learning needs made apparent by his work with a problem. In this setting, the teacher's role can be seen as that of a guide or facilitator. To perform this role, the teacher needs to be aware of the clinical reasoning process and willing to allow the student to learn by his own experimentation, inquiry, and study. He must be allowed to learn by mistakes. The teacher serves as both a monitor and stimulus to the process by asking leading questions, challenging thinking, and raising issues or points that need to be considered. In all of this, he attempts to help them help themselves in the educational process.

Problem-Based Learning with Other Problem Formats

The same basic interactive process can be used with other problem formats. Some, such as the PMP, SMP, and the P4, are designed to facilitate the application by the student of clinical reasoning skills by simulating the real clinical challenge through the presentation of a brief initial picture of the patient's problem as it would have occurred in real life. The student is asked to look at the initial cues presented, form an initial concept about the problem, produce early hypotheses, choose an inquiry path to develop a problem formulation, and refine his hypotheses. In the same manner, the teacher can stimulate thinking and help shape student reasoning processes through questions and discussions at appropriate points in work with the problem, as was done during the "time out" sessions with the simulated patient.

The PMP restricts the student to limited initial choices after the initial problem exposition. This prevents a free choice of all possible actions by the students. As mentioned previously, this tends to cue the student and limits the application of inquiry strategies to the student's hypotheses. The PMP does allow the student to follow the progress of the case, however, and to make decisions about laboratory tests, results of laboratory tests, treatment programs, and follow-up evaluations. The SMP allows the student to decide on his own actions at many points in his work with the patient problem but he is unable to follow the consequences of his own inquiry. He must follow the particular evaluation and treatment sequence carried out by those responsible for the actual patient or by the designers of the problem. This can be valuable if there is no teacher working with the student, since he cannot go off bravely into blind alleys or inappropriate activities as he follows the problem sequence. With the SMP, the student can compare his own thinking and actions with those revealed in the problem. The PMP and the P4, however, allow the students to follow the consequences of their own actions and learn by trial and error.

The printed case history cannot be used, as it is, to develop problem-based learning. It has to be segmented by the teacher before being given to the students so that it can be presented in a manner similar to the SMP. As another alternative, the students can cover the printed problem with a sheet of paper and slowly expose sequences of the text, treating each sequence as in the SMP format by deciding on their hypotheses, formulations, and actions at each point and then revealing another bit of the text to see what was actually done in the patient problem. Unfortunately, the text of the usual printed case history is not organized in the manner that makes this approach as effective as it might be. Such case histories can be rewritten by the teacher or a student so that they present in a manner that more closely simulates the way the actual patient may have presented. If the teacher is a clinician who has had experience with patient problems in the same area as the students are studying, he can present patient problems to them verbally. With his expertise, he can choose to present it in the manner of an SMP or a P4. As always, *the choice depends upon the educational goals.*

Outside of the simulated patient or real patient, the P4 and certain computer simulations are the only problem formats in which the student can interact with the problem in a way that allows free choice of actions in his inquiry strategy. As a consequence, these formats most closely simulate the challenge of the real clinical setting. They do not require a teacher to be present to provide the data at each step. In addition, because these formats are standardized, evaluation can be made of the student's performance against the performance of peers or professionals who have also worked with the problem. In all of these problem formats, students should be able to continue and follow the patient's problem over time, to choose tests and investigations, and to see the results of these investigations. The student should be able to decide on treatment and see the response of the patient to these decisions. The availability of X rays, scans, patient images, electrocardiographs, electro-encephologram, biopsy specimens, consultative reports, and the like enhance skills of observation and interpretation.

The Use of Patients

As the students become more adept in their clinical reasoning processes, the interruptions for discussion and analysis can be less and less frequent. At times it might be valuable for one student to carry through the evaluation of the patient problem to the end, with critique by his peers and teacher when he is finished. Once the student has acquired some basic skills in clinical reasoning and examination in his encounters with any of the simulation formats mentioned, he should have repeated opportunities to apply this learning to encounters with real patients. This reinforces his learning and provides incentives for more learning, since the patient experience almost always will raise many unanswered questions. With patients, the student group cannot take "time out" to discuss the usual initial concepts, hypotheses, formulations, underlying pathogenic mechanisms, and treatment possibilities. For many patients, such discussion could prove upsetting, if not demoralizing. Even if the group has agreed to select their words carefully and avoid discussions about disease processes and prognosis, slip-ups invariably occur in animated discussions. The patient easily misinterprets words and actions in his anxiety or concern about his medical problem. Although many faculty insist that this is not the case and such discussions can be handled around the patient without any problem, those who have looked carefully into the effect it has on the patient and his care in the hospital do not agree. In addition, these discussions often take too long and fatigue the patient, interfering with scheduled activities, tests, or the administration of treatment. Much of this activity, often done without concern for the patient, is unnecessary if other varieties of simulation can be used with the students. It is important that the patient experiences provided by teachers in medical schools be models of humane and caring attitudes if we are to expect these to be fostered in the medical student.

Nevertheless, a number of approaches are possible with student groups that capitalize on the opportunity provided by experience with real patients and complement learning from other problem-simulation formats. For example, one student can interview the patient while the rest observe. When he feels he has obtained the information he needs on history, other members of the group can be asked if they have any questions they would like to ask the patient. The teacher usually can guess the hypotheses and formulations implied by the student's questions and can keep notes on any questions or comments about the student's approach he may want to discuss later. If he has worked previously with the students on other simulation formats, he knows their habits and backgrounds and can interpret the actions they take with the patient. The students should keep similar notes about their own thoughts and observations and those of others during the patient encounter. After the first student has completed his interview with the patient and the other students have been given an opportunity to ask additional questions, another student is given the task of performing only the most appropriate physical examination items on the patient as the others watch. The student is given the challenge of performing only those examinations that are of the highest priority or value in establishing the correct hypotheses or diagnoses. This has the double advantage of keeping the patient encounter short and interesting as well as challenging the student's reasoning. Again, when he is finished, the other students are asked if there are any further examinations they would like to perform. The same observations are made during this part of the encounter. At the end, the teacher may wish to ask some questions of the patient and perform examination items for the students to observe and discuss subsequently. The students should guess why these particular items, in addition to what they have done already, are being performed for them by the teacher. In addition to demonstrating information that may have been missed, the teacher may have to repeat certain actions that already have been performed by the students, such as questions or examination items, if he feels the students need to see a different or better technique than the one that was used. This also can be done if he feels that the data obtained need further elaboration or clarification. In this format, all the students in the group can be asked, with permission from the patient, to examine fundi or repeat certain parts of the examination, especially if proprioceptive or tactile observations need to be made. The group can then retire to a room away from the patient and discuss the data base obtained, their hypotheses, the problem formulation, their concepts of altered anatomy or physiology, the treatment, progress, and so forth. The student also should have the challenge of eventually returning to the patient and explaining, at the patient's level, what has transpired, so that the patient is reassured about the encounter.

Developing Clinical Reasoning in Clinical and Postgraduate Years

A variation of this approach can be used by students in their clinical years or by house staff groups of any size to encourage further development of clinical reasoning skills. A student or house staff officer who has already performed a workup on the patient describes the patient's presenting picture and then asks members of the group to ask him questions as if he were the patient. In this approach, the thinking of the group members can be discussed while they attempt to evaluate the patient problem by the questions they ask. Whatever information the group may have requested that the presenter had not obtained from the patient is noted down for subsequent inquiry when the patient is brought into the room. At that time, another member of the group, who has never seen the patient previously, is asked to ask the unanswered questions and any other questions that the group may have identified as in need of further probing or clarification. This member of the group also is asked to perform an appropriate physical examination on the patient in front of the rest of the group. Again, he is asked to perform only those items of examination that are absolutely necessary to refine the formulations and hypotheses already developed by the group and not to bore the group with any routine examinations. This is a challenge in priority decision making and the ability to use the physical examination as a problem-oriented data-collecting tool. When this student has finished, the group is asked if they have any other items of examination they would like to see performed before the patient leaves. Their reason for these items can be discussed later when the patient leaves the room, at which point the member of the group who performed the physical examination (who had never seen the patient previously) is asked to discuss the case and identify his problem list and management plans. He also can be asked to identify the underlying pathophysiology in the particular case and to describe the subsequent workup he would propose. If any of the studies he would request, such as X rays, are available they can be presented for interpretation by another member of the group and incorporated into the ongoing evaluation and treatment of the patient. The examiner, the second student to work with the patient, has to defend his thinking against questions and challenges by the original student or the house staff officer who had worked up the patient. Presumably, this latter person has already done some study of the literature or had consultation with staff and has a more extensive knowledge base about the patient's problem. This can be a powerful method for refining clinical reasoning and promoting further learning about patient problems on a group basis. This approach can be extended to incorporate self-study and evaluation.

The students' clinical reasoning skills can be developed further in their clinical work by applying the pressure of time to force them to eliminate irrelevant, time-consuming questions or examinations. This is accomplished by insisting that patient encounters be completed in less and less time. If their prior workup of a new patient took one hour, then they are required to complete the next new patient encounter in forty-five minutes. At the same time, the teacher insists on even more rigorous problem formulation, diagnostic decisions, and management plans. This permits the students to employ only the most relevant actions, questions, and examinations with the highest payoff with regard to finding the patient's problem. This simulates an important aspect of the real-life task that students will face as physicians: they will have patient responsibilities that exceed the time that they have available to carry them out. A subsequent, brief review by the teacher of the patient examined by the student will reveal the precision of the students' reasoning and their use of clinical skills. It is a continual source of amazement how effective this pressure, deliberately applied in the clinical setting, is in forging secure and confident clinical reasoning skills. Despite the students' initial protest at the discomfort of pressure, they soon find themselves moving to a new level of performance associated with condifence and skills that appear to be innate and easy. The analogy of this approach to training athletes, musicians, and others who must master complex skills is apparent.

Changes in Student Reasoning Associated with Learning

As teachers work with students through the undergraduate curriculum, facilitating their clinical reasoning process with a variety of simulations and real patients, changes can be seen in their clinical reasoning that signify progress toward the skills required of the physician. There are some tendencies for harmful changes in the student's clinical reasoning process, however, that are a consequence of his growing sophistication in medical knowledge and facts, as well as increasing experiences with patients. When students first enter medical school, they are not inhibited by specific medical knowledge and, therefore, tend to be more creative in their generation of hypotheses and tend to produce hypotheses which are relatively nonspecific. As their medical knowledge increases and they become increasingly aware of specific disease states and disorders, as well as aware of the vastness of medical information that they do not know, their tendency to produce multiple hypotheses decreases, yet their skills in vertical thinking improve. Their increasing knowledge base allows them to develop better methods for eliminating or ranking hypotheses and obtaining data that can support or weaken hypotheses. Unfortunately, this can lead to a situation where the students begin to process one hypothesis at a time because they have become so restricted in the formation of multiple hypotheses. Frequently, the teacher has to liberate their thinking by such tricks as saying, "Imagine that you are not in medical school but out in the street and we are casually discussing a patient problem like this; what ideas might occur to you as being responsible for this patient's problem?" Maneuvers such as this tend to produce increased freedom in developing hypotheses about the problem. Another tendency in medically sophisticated students is to make hypotheses that are too specific and confined. As mentioned in an earlier chapter, hypotheses that are too narrow or too specific tend to become less adaptable to change as new data appear; oftentimes they prevent the student from realizing that there are data that would suggest alternative hypotheses or a modification in the hypotheses that they are carrying in their heads. Students also tend to apply facts that they have recently learned about patients or diseases or to apply techniques that they have just learned about interview or examination, without concern for their applicability or appropriateness to the problem at hand. In other words, they perform something because they know how to do it, not because it seems particularly relevant. Another tendency can be called "eureka" thinking, in which the student recognizes a symptom or sign that has been considered pathognomonic for a particular disease and goes ahead to prove that this is what the patient has, without carefully questioning other alternatives. Another mistake in the same line is the tendency to force the patient's problem to fit a pattern the student has just learned about a disease or a disorder. These problems need to be considered with regard to the teacher's activities in shaping the student's problem-solving development.

The teacher should always insist that the students develop multiple hypotheses. These hypotheses should be as nonspecific as possible until the data suggest a more specific focus. Hypotheses should form a "ring" or net that catches all the data from the patient; simultaneous processing of the hypotheses should be facilitated so as to increase the efficiency and effectiveness of the clinical reasoning process. Hypotheses should be developed that concern management at a later stage in the interaction with the patient problem. In addition, the teacher should be certain that the students develop an increasing awareness of payoff factors in the patient's management, that is, those things that will meet more effectively the patient's needs as opposed to treating the specific disorder at hand. At the same time, he should be certain that the students continue to accept more responsibility for the evaluation and care of the patient they are dealing with, that they develop an increasing awareness of disease prevalence and disease treatability as payoff factors and management decisions, and that they develop an appropriate balance of concern between psychosocial and medical problems. The students should be helped to accept ambiguity in analyzing patient problems. They must learn to cope with incomplete data in making decisions and to accept the fact that there may be multiple right paths, with no one right answer, in working with a patient problem. It is important that such problems be put deliberately into learning formats.

CHAPTER 6

Facilitating Self-Directed Study in Problem-Based Learning: Continued Skills for the Teacher and Student

Any patient problem in medicine can lead the student into a study of many subject areas or disciplines. The most profitable subject areas are those in which the student finds his knowledge and understanding weak or lacking. For the beginning student, this approach could conceivably lead to almost a year's study, encompassing all the new knowledge relevant to his learning needs in areas such as anatomy, physiology, biochemistry, pathology, pharmacology, epidemiology, clinical skills, and medicine. A focus is needed to restrict study to the most appropriate areas and to determine the depth or extent of study in the areas selected.

Educational Prescription

Making an educational prescription helps both the student and the student group develop a focus for study. The educational prescription is a personal statement of educational intent that is drawn up by the student as a reference for decision making about appropriate study with any problem. Properly constructed, it allows the student to combine his own educational objectives with the objectives of the school and the particular section of the curriculum he is in at any particular time. This, combined with the results of his work on any particular problem, allows him to determine an appropriate plan for study. As time goes on and the student gets a clearer concept of his career objectives in medicine and the education needed to meet these objectives, the educational prescription can undergo any number of mid-course corrections. It should be considered a navigational aid in mapping a course through medical school and beyond. This educational prescription also serves as a commitment by the student, and can be used by both the student and the teacher as a reference for evaluation of the student's progress. The combined educational prescription of the students in a working group allows both students and the teacher to be aware of the particular individual resources in knowledge and experience that exist for each member in the group. It also allows the students to realize each other's specific educational needs so that study plans of the group can be designed to meet these individual needs. Each member can see where he might assist others in the group with particular educational needs that relate to an area in which he may have experience or background.

The formality of an educational prescription can vary widely, all the way from a detailed contract with a specific structure, as advocated by Knowles (1975) to a brief, informal discussion by a group experienced in self-evaluation and self-directed study. It seems important, however, for the student to commit himself to paper. This forces the student to consider many factors important in his education and to be specific about his study priorities, and allows the effectiveness of the educational prescription as a self-evaluation and self-study tool to be assessed. The educational prescription has the following components.

1. It should incorporate the overall educational goals or objectives of the school, if known or stated.

2. It should express the educational objectives of that portion of the curriculum or the specific course in which the student is presently studying. If these are not stated, the teacher should be asked to provide them. If this is not possible, they can be deduced from an available description of the course content and/or the makeup of the final examination in prior years, if known. If none of these can be found, the student must guess what they are from whatever cues are available.

3. It should contain a statement of the student's particular strengths in knowledge and skills, related to the present area of study, by virtue of background experiences or prior education. The students may have been involved in hobbies, summer employment, undergraduate studies, or graduate work before medical school in areas of basic or clinical health science, or may have been involved in related professional health work. As the student progresses through school, this list grows to include prior medical studies, as well as elective and extra-curricular activities, such as clinics, field work, or research.

4. The student's specific learning objectives should be stated, in light of his present concept of his probable career in medicine. Many teachers feel

that the student is not capable of making these decisions early in his medical school years, at least not until he is well into his clinical years. This is probably not true. On reflection, most students find they could have focused on their careers at a very early stage. They have clear feelings about the possibility of such alternatives as family practice, pediatrics, psychiatry, or surgery. They also have some feelings about the possibility of private or group practice, as opposed to institutional or academic settings, or whether research is of interest. The accuracy of these objectives is not of great importance in the early years; the exercise of thinking about a future course is important. As students progress in their education and gain experience or exposure to different areas of medicine, career objectives will become more and more specific and accurate. Even the vaguest objectives are helpful to the educational prescription. If for example, the student feels he will never be a psychiatrist, then study in the psychiatric or psychosocial aspects of patient problems should be sought by this student, since his postgraduate training may not provide a foundation in these areas. If the student knows that a rural practice in family medicine is likely, then he would want to ensure that he is well versed in those aspects of the relevant basic sciences and clinical sciences that are most important for this type of practice. When the student is in doubt, a discussion with a member of the faculty regarding his tentative career would help him sort out priorities for study.

The student, with the help from peers or teacher if appropriate, should draw up his educational prescription for the particular course, curricular unit, elective experience, clinic or whatever educational setting he is entering. The prescription can have the following additional components.

1. School objectives personalized by the student so that they are relevant to his concept of the behaviors or competencies he should be able to demonstrate on graduation (see Chapter 1).

2. Course objectives or guidelines that describe the behaviors or competencies the student feels he should be able to demonstrate on the completion of the particular course, unit, clinic, or elective with which he is involved. If the type of evaluation provided by the school or teacher at the completion will not measure his attainment of this stated objective, the student might consider how he could satisfy himself that they have been met. Chapter 7 describes the evaluation techniques that match specific educational objectives.

3. Subject or skill areas that need to be emphasized in studies and applied to his work with the problem encountered. Those that may have been neglected so far in his education, or represent high priorities for his career goals as seen at this particular time, are especially important.

4. Subject areas or skills that may have received sufficient emphasis in past studies and could be avoided profitably in the interest of time management, even if the problems encountered may suggest more intriguing aspects for study in these areas.

These study plans can be discussed within working groups, with input by peers and the teacher, so that an overall stragety can be designed for the group that could best meet individual needs.

These educational prescriptions can be used as a means to determine which problems should be selected next for study by the individual students or group. A range of problems or units are available and the students are free to develop their own sequence. The teacher, or a student selected in rotation, can be given the task of reviewing the available problems and selecting the ones more suited to the group's objectives. If the problems are prescribed by the teacher or faculty for the student in a particular course, or if they are selected randomly, the educational prescription will ensure that students decide on appropriate self-directed study.

At this point, it should be obvious that the faculty can ensure that the scope or focus of learning is adequate, through the selection and range of problems offered to the student.

Educational Issues

As the student or students work with a problem format, simulated patient or patients, they should keep the segments of their clinical reasoning process attuned to their educational prescription. If basic mechanisms and learning in basic science are the goals, the hypotheses developed should attempt to describe the range of possibilities, in altered anatomy, physiology, biochemistry, psychology, or pharmacology, as mechanisms to explain the problem. The hypotheses should describe the range of possible pathological mechanisms, if this is the learning goal. They should describe the possible diseases, disorders, or syndromes and treatment approaches, if clinical science learning is the goal. Not infrequently, multiple levels of learning are identified and the hypotheses may have to be made from several different areas in sequence. For example, initial hypotheses may refer to anatomical or physiological concepts. When the appropriate concept has been decided upon, hypotheses concerning pathological mechanisms can be considered. Finally, if appropriate to educational objectives, hypotheses regarding diseases or syndromes can be used to arrive at a clinical diagnostic formulation. At all stages of this process, however, the students should ask themselves:

1. Do the hypotheses raised suggest study into one or more specific areas or disciplines?
2. What questions have been raised in working with this problem that cannot be answered and suggest the need for study?
3. What data are needed to define the problem further, select more appropriate hypotheses, or develop new hypotheses?
4. Do I have sufficient background knowledge or skills to continue working with this problem?

Notes should be taken regarding the study areas and unanswered questions raised by either the individual student or by a student acting on behalf of a group or class of students.

If the answer to the last question in the previous list is "yes," further work with the problem is possible. If the answer is felt to be "no," then the following possibilities need to be reviewed.

1. If the student's or students' knowledge is felt to be insufficient in areas related to the problem but this does not hamper further reasoning or progress, then the study issues or unanswered questions can be written down for later review.

2. If the student or students feel that their knowledge is definitely insufficient in an important area but that the answers needed could be acquired easily and quickly by using a resource immediately at hand, they can stop to review the resource and then continue on with the problem. Note of the issues studied should be made, however, in case further study may seem warranted later, in light of the ultimate outcome with the problem. Such convenient resources are texts, monographs, journals at hand, or faculty nearby who could answer a brief, well-focused question.

3. If the student or students feel that their knowledge is insufficient to continue with the problem and that the needed information is going to take prolonged study, then they should stop and decide upon a self-study program.

4. If the student or students feel that their knowledge is insufficient in an area directly related to subjects or skills that the educational prescription indicates need to be emphasized, then it might be most profitable to stop at this point and decide on a self-study program so that this new knowledge can be applied back to the problem after it has been acquired.

If the students are able to continue with the problem without taking a major break for self study before their work with the problem has been concluded, they can proceed to evaluate their work with the problem before drawing up a study plan (see Chapter 7). At the conclusion of the problem, they should write a problem formulation or diagnosis and a treatment plan, if clinical goals were implied in their work. If their goals or objectives were primarily in basic science areas, they could write up a final statement of the underlying pathological mechanisms responsible for the problem and how they might be corrected. This formulation, as well as a review of their initial approach to the problem, can be evaluated against what they have finally learned about the problem. Their approach with the problem, questions asked, physical examination items performed, tests performed, interpretation of tests, management, and so forth can be evaluated against the discovered outcome with the problem or with any evaluation materials that have been supplied with the problem. They can ask questions about the adequacy or appropriateness of their initial cues and concepts, their hypotheses, and their sequence of actions. Did they go down a blind alley in their reasoning? Were the assumed pathological mechanisms correct? Were the proposed treatment plans appropriate in terms of the final outcome? And so forth. These all can be reviewed and, in turn, can lead to a list of appropriate areas of study or to the acquisition of necessary knowledge or skills related to their deficiencies in the problem and their educational prescription.

To summarize at this point, the students always must be aware of possible educational issues raised in their ongoing work with a problem, against the background of an educational prescription. Although work in self-directed study itself occurs after the application of clinical reasoning skills to the problem, the information base needed for self-directed study is obtained as the students work with the problem. This self-directed study phase starts whenever active, ongoing work with the problem stops. This is true regardless of whether it occurs somewhere in the middle of the problem or at its conclusion. In turn, when the second phase of self-directed study ends, the information gained by the study must be applied back to the problem to complete it, to analyze how effectively it was handled, and to determine what has been learned. This must become a lifetime habit that the student, as a physician, will continue to use in his work with patient problems, allowing him to update his knowledge as he continues to work.

Study Plans

The questions raised during work with the problem, the specific educational tasks raised by the nature of the problem, and the difficulties the problem presents to the student or students are all noted down on paper and then reviewed in terms of the educational prescription. As a consequence, specific areas that need to be studied or specific experiences or skills that need to be gained can be put into priority, converting the recorded list into a study plan. This priority listing should be concerned with the depth and focus of the study. For example, if they had dealt with a hereditary or familial disorder of the nervous system, the student or students would have to determine whether the genetics of that particular problem need to be studied or whether some background in neurological genetics might be reviewed briefly, depending upon their background knowledge and the priority of other educational issues facing them. In all of this, the teacher should provide guidance to the students through the issues or questions he raises during the design of their study plan. The teacher raises issues that may have been overlooked and challenges the priorities established by the students, once again applying the same teaching skills used during their reasoning with the problem.

The next question facing the student or student group, with or without the teacher, is in regard to the learning resources that should be used to gain the information and skills required.

In this text, the terms "student," "students," and "teacher" seem to be intermixed. The problem-based learning skills described can be used by a group of students with a teacher, by a group of students without a teacher, or by individual students on their own individualized study program. These processes also can be used within a class working on the same problem. As this approach applies to a variety of educational settings at a variety of levels, the specific usage of these procedures would vary among these combinations as dictated by the students' skills, their confidence in their clinical reasoning and self-study process, ant the curricular design. These approaches are certainly not limited to undergraduate medicine, they are perfectly applicable to postgraduate studies and other health-professional education programs. Again, it's worth reviewing the fact that these processes of clinical reasoning and self-directed study can be applied with any variety of problem, whether it has been specifically designed as a problem format (PMP, SMP, P4, computer), a simulated patient, a case history, or a real patient.

Learning Resources

There is a variety of learning resources available to students. This term is not used in a restricted sense here; it designates any resource that the student can use to gain needed information, experience, or skills. The asterisks in the following list designate those resources that usually are available to the practicing physician.

1. *Printed formats*
    *a. Books: Texts, manuals, guides, monographs, seminars

      *b. Journals: Investigations, reviews, editorials
     *c. Reprints
      d. Syllabi
  2. *Audiovisual formats*
      a. Slide-tape productions
    *b. Videotapes
    *c. Audiotapes
      d. Slide collections
      e. Films
  3. *Models and specimens* include plastic, plaster, mechanical, gross and microscopic specimens, cadavers, prepared slices, and imbedded specimens
  4. *People*
      a. Teaching faculty: Clinical, basic science, other university departments
      b. Research faculty
    *c. Specialists: Medicine, nursing, other health professions
      d. Administrators
      e. Other students: Medicine, nursing, health professions, others at a university
      f. Community
    *g. Peers
  5. *Places*
      a. Clinics
      b. Wards
      c. Laboratories: Research, clinical
      d. Community agencies
      e. Field studies
      f. Health projects

Experience over the years with a problem-based, self-study, student-centered curriculum at McMaster University medical school has shown that printed materials and faculty are the most commonly used resources for study, despite the availability of a large number of audiovisual materials, models, and specimens. Since the asterisked items are the resources our students will have available after graduation for continuing their education, it is particularly important that they develop secure skills in using them during their undergraduate education. Problem-based learning will facilitate these skills if the student is continuously required to obtain information of all varieties, from the library, printed resources, physicians, students, peers, or colleagues. He will learn the more effective and efficient approaches in gaining this information from these sources. Again, this is an area where the teacher can be helpful in his guidance.

Dimensions other than the availability in community settings need to be considered in the selection of a learning resource, such as the following.

1. How contemporary and accurate is the information? How would you rank the following items as to the "freshness" of the information they offer: textbook, journal, review article, faculty information, audiovisual resource?

2. Is the information too broad or superficial, or is it too focused, detailed, or specific?

3. How easily can the specific area of information desired for study be found? Can it be found without the student being exposed to unwanted information or becoming involved in time-consuming activities? For example, have you tried finding a specific piece of information in a film, videotape, audiotape, or a slide-tape show?

4. How long does it take to acquire the information during study? The student usually can acquire far more information in less time by reading than he can by hearing a tape or listening to a conversation.

5. Can the information be reviewed easily, to refresh memory or to correlate the information with other sources of information?

6. Is the information resource easy to find and use? Is it portable? These characteristics allow the student to study from the resource, at any time and in any place.

7. Is the medium that is used the best one to transmit the information the student wishes to acquire. For example, if the subject under study relates to motion, such as patient movement or examination procedure, then a videotape or film would probably be the best medium to transmit that information. If the student should look at or manipulate something at the same time he receives the information, then audiotape has distinctive advantages. If the phenomenon to be studied is spatial or three-dimensional, a model may be the best medium. If seeing or feeling is important, then clinical or surgical experience may be best. If abstract concepts of categories of information need to be acquired, certainly the printed word or a conversation will do this best.

These criteria are important for effective and efficient self-study and reveal why books, journals, peers, and faculty are most commonly used as resources. They are convenient, most up-to-date, easily found, easily accessible, and the exact information needed can be located without having to wade through everything else. Printed works have a variety of systems that allow information to be found easily through published indexes, annual reviews, and tables to contents. It is easy for a student to scan or read in detail printed material, depending upon his objectives. It is also important, nevertheless, for the student to gain skills necessary to manipulate and utilize videotapes, audiotape players, projectors, slide-tape machines, and other media monsters, since he will have to use them in many instances in the future and this mechanical knowledge will save him considerable time and frustration. The use of experiences in clinics, agencies, or projects is an often neglected area of study; however, these settings may represent the best way to learn the skills of interview, examination, and observation, and the use and interpretation of tests in specialized areas.

Learning Style

The most valuable aspect of self-study is that it allows the student to learn in the manner he feels is most natural for him or in which he learns best. If the student has never thought about this, it might be valuable for him to reflect on his past learning and how he thinks he learns most effectively. For example, does the student

1. Read, then summarize his reading with notes or diagrams?
2. Read and underline or make marginal notes?
3. Take notes or make diagrams on separate paper, as he reads, and then summarize his reading in written form?
4. Read and then discuss what has been read with someone else?
5. Read and then dictate his thoughts into an audiotape for later replay and study?
6. Read and make flash cards of important points to review?
7. Feel he learns better by listening to lectures, tapes, and discussions that he does by reading?
8. Learn best if he tries to teach someone or debate with someone about what he has learned?

An awareness of the options available in study and experimentation can be helpful. There are many educators who feel that the often voiced concerns that resources should be made available in a variety of formats to accommodate different learning styles may be overdone. The important thing is for the student to find the right resources for the information or skills needed and to have a study technique that allows him to make the most of this resource. Conventional concerns in this area may not be as applicable in the problem-based learning format, since the information acquired by the student will be actively applied back to his work with the problem, reinforcing what has been learned and allowing him to consider this information in perhaps a different way than just memorizing what he has read or listened to.

Another valuable aspect of self-directed learning is that the student can take the time necessary for him to learn. Since all students have different backgrounds, different knowledge, and experience bases, as well as different styles and abilities in learning, the speed and depth of study is a very individual matter. As we are concerned here with the quality of learning in the education of physicians, we would like to be certain that fundamentals are mastered at each point so that more advanced concepts and new knowledge can be built on these fundamentals at any time. The constraint of time should be dropped from the student's learning process. As all students will encounter both difficult and easy areas of learning, even though they may be different for each student, a group of students on a self-study program will probably end up taking rather similar amounts of time in their overall studies. The important factor is that the student, in self-directed study, can budget his time, review, repeat, ponder, and skim, as needed for his own learning. Even in a class-oriented, teacher-centered program, adequate self-study time can enhance the learning process.

It might be worth considering where this self-directed study approach should be classified in the teaching–learning options described in Chapter 1. Working with a problem by applying evolving clinical reasoning skills is certainly problem-based learning, as is the selection of learning issues that results from this work. The study plan, however, is a guide to subject-based learning. The learning resources are invariably subject-oriented in their content. The study questions and issues usually are devoted to areas or disciplines in clinical or basic science. Content is being learned, discipline and subject areas are being studied, and the student is gaining knowledge. The difference is that *the student has identified the need for his learning,* sees its relevance, wants to learn, and will *apply it back to the problem,* the focus of his professional skills. This is a point that often is not understood clearly by teachers who feel that problem-based learning somehow means the students do not learn the facts of important subjects or disciplines in medicine.

Returning to the Problem

Several crucial steps in self-directed study or learning still lie ahead. Now that the student or students have completed their self-prescribed studies to their own satisfaction, they are ready to return to the problem. With a group of students, the time to return to the problem might have been agreed upon in advance or prescribed in their course. With the individual student, it may occur whenever the student feels ready. The approach used can be highly individual but the crucial ingredient is that the information is applied back to work with the problem. It would be a serious mistake for the students to assume that the information or skills they learned in their study have made the problem understandable and that, because they now know the underlying mechanism, or what questions should have been asked, or what diagnosis really should have been made, or what the treatment should have been, they can continue with another problem. If the self-directed study occurred in the middle of the problem because the student or students ran into a major problem in knowledge, then it is less of a danger, for they will pick up where they have left off with that problem and utilize the newly gained information to continue with their reasoning. If the self-directed study occurred after the problem was completed, however, the students may feel that all questions have been cleared up and they can move on to the next problem. In this instance, they should review the steps in their clinical reasoning from the start, now that they have become more knowledgeable, touching on the following points.

1. What initial cues should have been noted and how should they have been interpreted?
2. What would have been an appropriate array of hypotheses as a guide to evaluating the problem?
3. How could the blind alleys or inefficient lines of inquiry in their investigation of the problem have been avoided?
4. Should the evolving and final problem formulation have been different?
5. What would have been the appropriate investigation or tests to use with that problem and in what sequence?
6. What were the mechanisms of altered form and function involved in the problem? Were they correctly identified?
7. Was the treatment plan or method of resolving the problem selected rational? Did it address itself to the underlying disease mechanisms or payoff concerns of the patient?
8. Were the relevant psychosocial concerns identified and handled appropriately?
9. What modifications in clinical skills, interview technique, physical examination, or interpersonal skills might have been useful?

The review of the individual steps in the clinical reasoning employed and the specific questions asked depend on the educational prescription and the study plan. A revised case write-up might be in order, for comparison to an initial problem list, diagnostic impression, or treatment plan. (The next chapter will continue with methods of formal or informal evaluation that might be used by students to assess their abilities and knowledge at this point.)

If the self-directed study occurred in the middle of the problem, another study period might occur at completion, to clean up some of the unfinished educational issues raised by the remainder of the work with the problem. However, the student or students could carry out the same review as described above even when they work uninterrupted to the conclusion of the problem.

Considering What Has Been Learned

The last, most neglected, and possibly most crucial step remains before self-study can be considered completed and evaluation or a new problem tackled. It is to *formalize* and *integrate* what has been learned at the completion of the problem episode. This must be done if the students are to capitalize fully on the educational advantage of problem-based learning. Studies performed by Schmidt (1965) and Hilgard (1953) clearly underline the need for students to take this step, if they are to maximize their ability to transfer what they have just learned to future problems. This requires the students to review their work with the problem and take stock of what has been learned and its significance. The following questions might be considered in doing this.

1. What principles or approaches have been learned in working with this problem that will help in work with future problems with similar characteristics?
2. What new information has been acquired in areas basic to medicine or in clinical medicine that enlarge upon, modify, or change the existing knowledge or understanding that the students have?
3. Can an outline, model, or generalization be made about the mechanisms or processes involved in this problem? For example, if an immunological reaction was involved, can the sequence of steps and factors involved be diagrammed? If resources in the community helped with the particular problem, can an outline be made of the resources available to patients in general and the ways in which they can be obtained?

Whatever approach is used, it is necessary that the students analyze, synthesize, and organize what has been learned and discuss how it might be applied to future problems.

This review is crucial not only to the learning of information in the clinical and basic sciences but to the development of clinical skills. For example, if the student works with a patient problem that features, among other things, muscle weakness, muscle atrophy, fasciculations, hypotonia, and decreased reflexes, he must be certain to fit these items together into a concept of lower motor neuron function and the trophic and control factors in neuronal function, neuromuscular transmission, and membrane excitability. As a result, the student will, more than likely, look for fasciculations on every patient he sees with muscle weakness, to see if motor neuron disorders might be present. Eventually, the student's search for fasciculations will become more effective and relevant as he automatically begins to focus the time-consuming search for fasciculation, confining it to patient problems in which the historical and physical data more strongly suggest the likelihood of motor neuron deficits. As a consequence, his brain will become programmed to recall motor neuron dysfunction as a possible hypothesis in any patient problem where this is a reasonable concern. His search for confirmatory signs or manifestations will become more relevant.

If possible, and if time permits, problems similar to the one just finished by the students could be undertaken to see if the skills, principles, and knowledge gained can be applied effectively to this new problem. It would be ideal if these could be real patients in which the learning could be transferred to the real world. In any case, a follow-up exercise used to recall and apply what has been learned in a slightly different context — be it a verbal presentation of a case by the teacher, a printed case history, a problem format, a simulated patient, or a real patient — will reinforce learning and recall of information and skills learned.

All of these steps for self-directed study, described in such detail, make the whole process seem like a complex, time-consuming ritual. As with the clinical reasoning process, however, most of this is a logical sequence of assessment of learning needs, formulation of a study plan, application of what has been learned to the problem, and assessment of what has been learned in general and its future implications. It soon becomes an almost-automatic and natural process. As in clinical reasoning, there are a few areas that need to be analyzed consciously in order to improve the effectiveness of this whole process. In self-directed learning, this involves a constant awareness of the educational prescription, the application of what has been learned back to the problem, and a final analysis and synthesis of what has been learned.

Evaluation in the Process of Self-Study

Self-evaluation complements self-study. Both the student and the physician must be able to determine the adequacy of their skills and knowledge, so that appropriate decisions can be made about future learning tasks and directions. The student needs to know how well he is accomplishing personal and school objectives. He needs to know if his educational prescription is effective and if he is moving on schedule toward the competencies he will need at graduation. The physician needs to know how well he is meeting the demands of his practice or the problems he confronts in his clinical or academic work.

The procedures described for facilitating or developing skills in clinical reasoning and self-study, in themselves, produce information that is evaluative; but it is informal in the sense that it is interwoven into the ongoing process of solving the patient problem. The students and teachers involved in this process certainly can get an accurate feeling about the adequacy of their skills and knowledge in dealing effectively with the problem and the issues at hand. More formal evaluation techniques need to be employed, however, to provide more effective overall assessment for both the students and teachers. This is the subject of the next chapter.

The Role of the Teacher in Problem-Based Learning

In this final section, we will consider more carefully the role of the teacher and the skills used by the teacher in problem-based learning. It is hoped that, at this point, the reader has already gained a feel for the teacher's behavior, as it is difficult to describe. The old oriental philosophy comes very close: "Give me a fish and I eat for a day; teach me to fish and I eat for a lifetime." The urge must be suppressed to tell the students what they should do in evaluating a problem properly or to give them the facts, principles, and concepts they need to understand the clinical challenges or related basic sciences involved. Faculty who are not comfortable with guiding students in the search for the right competencies and facts typically react by sitting by and becoming mute, letting the students say and do what they want. When teachers finally become exasperated with what seems to be time-wasting, incompetent wandering by students, "when so much has to be learned in medical school," they burst forth with criticisms of the student's work or lecture on the subject of the problem.

At the McMaster University Medical School, teachers were put with groups of students who were working in problem areas that were either unfamiliar to the teacher or were not in his area of expertise. This was deliberately designed to inhibit any tendency on the part of the teacher to lecture the students in his area of knowledge. Unfortunately, the basic concern of teachers who are uncomfortable with facilitating learning, as opposed to dispensing facts, is what they should do when the students are obviously way off the track in their reasoning or bring incorrect information to work with the problem. If they are teaching an area in which they are not an expert, this worry is escalated into panic by the concern that they won't even know when the students are off base or incorrect in their information. This use of the "non-expert" teacher also prevents the students from having a faculty re-source ready to answer questions, which might allow the group to deal more effectively with the problem at hand. This, of course, requires the expert to know when it would be more appropriate for the students not to receive a direct answer to a simple question but to find the information on their own. This experiment thus showed that it is far better to have an expert working with the students, one who knows if the students are in a quandary or are going down the wrong track; but who also knows how to get them to discover this for themselves, to learn by making mistakes, and to reason their way to the right conclusions. Such an expert can provide the students with better evaluative feedback about their learning, relevant to their own objectives.

This approach of the teacher also has been described incorrectly as the teacher becoming another member of the group and learning along with the students, all being equals. If this were so, why would one bother to provide a teacher? One might as well put another real student in there, who should be learning along with the group. This is not to imply that the teacher doesn't learn in the process; quite the contrary. When the students try their own approach and dig after their own information about the problem, the teacher is constantly enriched with fresh ways to look at problems and with new information; however, in this learning method the teacher is the guide, the captain of the team, and is responsible to the school for ensuring that the students are provided every opportunity to learn. The conventional "teacher up there" and "student down there" relationship merely inhibits the adult, responsible learning expected of the student and stifles the openness about their thinking that is required if improvement of individual skills and knowl-edge is to occur. The teacher in problem-based learning is an expert in the group who has been given the responsibility of helping the students to learn. He must know the structure of clinical reasoning and self-directed study and must guide the students' work and self-evaluation through these sequences, making sure that learning is adequate and sound.

People learn by doing and by discovering their own mistakes. The teacher in problem-based learning allows this to occur. At the same time, he encourages the students to apply sound reasoning skills in their work with a problem and to use effective study skills in acquiring the knowledge appro-priate to their needs or objectives. He also ensures that they apply this knowledge in their work with other problems.

A common concern of faculty attempting this approach is what they should do when they see students making mistakes. If they don't outright tell the students that they are wrong, what should they do when they see them

1. Drawing wrong conclusions?
2. Not thinking of the correct alternatives?

3. Being superficial in the probing of the problem?
4. Going nowhere in their work with the problem?
5. Providing incorrect explanations for the phenomenon they are observing or considering?
6. Giving wrong information?
7. Doing inappropriate study?

The options for the teacher are endless. The following are suggested comments that could be modified to suit any of the situations just listed.

1. "Why did you come to that conclusion? Could there be another alternative?"
2. Turn to a student other than the one talking and ask, "Do you agree with what he just said?" (Usually, in time, the teacher learns the background and personality of the students well enough to use this ploy with deadly accuracy, knowing what student can be relied upon to make certain comments.)
3. "If what you say is true, then how would you explain . . . ?" (Give the students an example of something related to the issue under discussion but which cannot be understood by the explanation they have just given.)
4. "With this kind of problem, have you ever thought about . . . ?"
5. "Are you satisfied with your explanations (hypotheses, alternatives, formulations) or are there other issues you need to consider?"
6. "Please explain what you have just said so that I can understand your statement (opinion, conclusions)."

Through all of this, the teacher has acted in the capacity of a guide. Although he has suggested he does not agree or he is concerned that the students are not on the right track, they still have to get to it on their own. Further discussion of the issues at hand or re-examination of their thinking caused by such comments will lead to better results. In addition, the student may not want to face the weaknesses of his logic or information; such challenges will force him to bring this to light so that better learning can occur. To ensure that such comments do not become a sure signal for wrong thinking or wrong information, the teacher should use the same questions when the student's actions or conclusions seem to be correct. Challenge them to explain or defend their thinking. If, for example, there really are no further alternatives to be considered, the first question still could be asked to see if the students realize this fact. Sometimes, under such a challenge, the students may produce some alternatives that the teacher may never have thought about.

Stronger ammunition sometimes is needed, yet it can be given in a manner that still puts learning responsibility on the student, such as the following.

1. "Are you sure of what you are saying?"
2. "Do you feel you need to look that point up?"
3. "You seem unsure. Could this be a learning issue that should be studied before we go further?"
4. "Perhaps there are better ways to examine this problem. Is there a resource that might be consulted?"
5. "I'm not sure you are right. Why don't you look that up and review it with us next time?" (Use this one most sparingly.)

As an information source, the teacher should respond to direct inquiry from the students only after he is sure they have exhausted their own logic or information base and feels that the information provided will facilitate further work with the problem at the time, without sacrificing the value of self-study.

The skills of the teacher in problem-based learning do not relate as much to his ability to dispense his knowledge and understanding as an expert in the areas of science or medicine as they do to his ability to help the student develop skills in scientific reasoning, self-study and self-evaluation. This analysis of the steps involved in facilitating clinical reasoning and self-directed study give the teacher a *structure* for the development of these skills that he or she can use as a guide in teaching.

Summary

In summary, the essential ingredients for this teaching approach are (1) a set of objectives which provide guidelines to the student in his selection of problems and areas of study, (2) an appropriately designed problem, and (3) a teacher who understands the process of clinical reasoning and is skilled in facilitating learning. The objectives usually will be a combination of the non-negotiable objectives identified by the school and the personal objectives of the student. Examples of well-designed problems are the P4 unit or the simulated patient. A competent teacher can guide students indirectly while they are actively involved in work with the problem simulation, stopping them at crucial points to ask about their thinking; why they asked the questions they did; their concept of the patient's problem; their guesses or hypotheses and how their actions relate to these; and how they are going to rank, refine, or eliminate hypotheses. The teacher should be able to promote discussion, retrials, and critiques among students. At all times, the teacher must be aware of the skills that he is trying to develop and shape in the student. The teacher should be able to diagnose the problems students are having in their use of the problem-solving process and ease them into increasingly sophisticated performances in which the student also develops an awareness of the effects of conscious and unconscious misperceptions or translation errors in converting the patient's words into the wrong medical term. He can help them develop concerns about payoff, likelihood, treatability, and awareness of the "whole" patient and his environment. This process ensures a transfer of skills from the simulation to real patients. The teacher guides the students' identification of their learning needs, the way they meet these needs, and the skill with which they apply their learning to work with other problems in medicine. The teacher assists the student in developing priorities for learning by helping him use both personal and the program objectives. This approach provides the students with motivation, as well as confidence in their medical problem-solving abilities. It provides assurance to the teacher that the student is demonstrating competent problem-solving or clinical reasoning skills and is capable of effective learning as a continuous, lifelong process.

CHAPTER 7

Evaluation of Problem-Based Learning and Clinical Reasoning

In all teaching–learning situations, evaluation on an informal or almost intuitive basis always is present. This is particularly true in problem-based learning. As students struggle with a problem, their ability to meet its challenges is usually quite apparent. This is particularly true when the problem is taken on and discussed within a small group of students with a teacher acting as a facilitator of the learning process. Self-directed study requires the student to review his own work with the problem, to generate the questions and issues raised during that work. This is an evaluation. In their study, students often are able to realize how well they understood the problem. Later on, when students work with patients during their clinical years, present their cases to faculty, and write up their case records, they are able to get more information about their skills and knowledge relevant to that patient problem. In day to day work, therefore, students constantly produce information that helps them evaluate their present skills and understanding. This information often is ignored. To develop good skills in self-evaluation, the student must be consciously aware of the information he continually receives about his abilities. If he is in a noncompetitive environment where the attainment of grades is not a principal goal, it is far easier for the student to become sensitive to this rich evaluative information and correctly interpret its significance.

Whenever faculty work with students individually or in small groups, whether it is in the early years or the clinical years, they develop distinct "gut" reactions after a short contact with students. They can sense those students they feel are "good," "sharp," or "in no trouble" from those students they feel are "in difficulty," "have problems," or are "inadequate." These reactions are not unlike the first hypotheses generated by the clinician in his early contact with the patient. They are based on their past experiences with students, their awareness of what the students' behavior represents, and their particular knowledge of the field of study in which the students are involved. These feelings are not the sole province of the teacher, as fellow students develop similar feelings about their colleagues and, on many occasions, may be less deceived than the teacher about a colleague's ability. As a consequence of being in a competitive, grade-oriented, teacher-centered curriculum, many students have learned to cover inadequacies; these are behaviors that fellow students can detect or sense much more easily. In the open, small-group, no-grade learning system where there is no inter-student competition, the peers' "crap detector" can be used by the teacher and the group for constructive evaluation of students.

As we have said, all kinds of evaluative information is generated as students work with their problems. Much of this is at an intuitive level that can be likened to the behavior of a clinician faced with a problem. If the teacher or student were asked specifically to diagnose the existence of any educational problem, to measure it or to provide clear-cut evidence of its existence, or to specify its seriousness, he would have to make more inquiries, just as in the clinical situation. He would have to ask questions and perform tests to establish the exact nature and extent of the educational problem. This chapter reviews those methods of inquiry and their relevance to problem-based learning.

Even if the student feels he is doing well and the teacher is comfortable with the student's performance, this may not be enough. The skills and knowledge that the student needs to acquire are extensive and complex. The student needs to have an evaluation tool that will tell him that he is on course in his education and that there are no undetected problems that need attention.

The teacher needs to have measurement tools that will help him document the student's progress, either to produce a grade, mark, or preferably, a certification of a satisfactory performance in the course. Evaluation tools that provide a grade or certification of accomplishment for the student are called "summative" evaluations. They should certainly include specific statements about any of the student's particular strengths and weaknesses that need to be considered by both the student and his teacher in his further work. Evaluation tools that are used to provide the student with immediate feedback concerning his progress and that allow him to correct weaknesses or be assured of accomplishments are called "formative" evaluations. The information gained from these provides guidelines for corrective actions in his future study.

Evaluation tools also are needed by the faculty, to evaluate the adequacy of their instructional program. They need to know if there are common problems among the students that may reflect inadequacies in the curriculum or the teaching–learning approach that is being used. These tools also are needed to evaluate specific learning tools, techniques, audiovisual packages, and the like.

Educational diagnostic tools are needed to establish learning needs and provide guideposts for the student. At McMaster University Medical School, evaluation was for many years almost principally the result of very well-established small-group sessions where the student and the "tutor" openly discussed their own ideas and concerns about each student in the group on a recurrent, formative basis. This culminated in a periodic summary that went into each student's records as he moved to another section of the curriculum. These reports were of a pass–fail nature, including a structured written report. Despite this exceedingly valuable system, which provided the students with the opportunity to develop skills in self-evaluation and receive constructive criticism from others, there was always a distinct feeling of anxiety on the part of the students, year after year, that there wasn't any "hard" or more objective measurement that could be used to assure progress or lack of progress and detect unrecognized deficiencies.

Evaluation should be an integral part of the learning process, where it can give the student accurate feedback about his progress and indicate specific learning needs. Since the ultimate goal of self-directed learning is to make it a part of the student's professional life, the evaluation tools should be designed so that the student may use them himself. Because many of the evaluation tools used in problem-based learning may not be available to the students after graduation, evaluation tools must be designed to help the student develop his own approaches to self-evaluation, ones that he can continue with after graduation.

All evaluation tools, tests, and techniques measure different phenomena or competencies in the student. It is important that the technique or test selected be appropriately matched to the competency of behavior to be analyzed or measured (Mager, 1973). This is particularly true in problem-based learning, as much of the concern for student performance centers around the clinical reasoning process and related skills, and not necessarily around the content the student may have memorized or may be able to recall. This comment may seem self-evident; however, multiple-choice, true-false, or other objective examinations that test recall of information are used the world over, supposedly to certify the student's clinical competence. This occurs in medical-school examinations, licensing examinations, and specialty certifying examinations. The exclusive use of examinations that test recall of information as the only method to certify clinical competence assumes that encyclopedic retention of facts in some way correlates with clinical competency. There is a growing body of information that shows that this assumption cannot be made (Wingard & Williamson, 1973). As stated in previous chapters, the fact that the student knows something is no assurance that he knows when or how to use that information. The evaluations that are used in problem-based learning should be designed to measure those skills. The following is a brief review of the range of evaluation tools characteristically used, and also of those perhaps not so characteristically used, with a discussion of their advantages and disadvantages.

Characteristics of Evaluation Techniques and Tools

There are certain characteristics of all evaluation tools and techniques that need to be considered carefully whenever they are employed. They can be put under the following convenient headings.

Process versus Content

This distinction has been stressed many times. Content evaluation is concerned with the information, concepts, and principles the student has acquired in his memory banks and can bring forth by recognition, recall, or associations. This is not a pure distinction; some content evaluations may ask the student to process the data by such cognitive activities as abstracting, identifying similarities or differences, synthesizing or integrating the data, or analyzing the material that is being presented.

Process evaluation, on the other hand, is concerned with the student's ability to observe data, solve problems or show aspects of the clinical reasoning process, make clinical and therapeutic decisions, and the like.

Process versus Outcome

An analogy may serve well here. There are several conceivable ways in which one might be able to measure the skill of the archer. One could score his stance, the way he holds the bow, the way he pulls back the arrow, and the manner of his release. These would be process measurements. On the other hand, one could score his ability to hit the target with the arrows. This would be an outcome measurement.

Measurement in medicine is similar but not as straightforward. If you watch a student examine a patient or simulated patient, or review the videotape of such an encounter and score his interpersonal, interview, and examination skills, you are involved in process measurement. If you use videotape recall techniques or postpatient interviews and analyze the student's reasoning with a problem, you are still using process measurements. On the other hand, if you score the diagnostic formulation and treatment plan the student designs or writes up, you are measuring outcome. This, however, is not really the outcome measurement that parallels the one in the archer analogy. This outcome is analogous to looking at the force and direction of the arrow as it leaves the bow, knowing what force and direction are usually required to hit the target. It is only if you could measure the student's ability to actually manage the patient's problem or improve the patient's condition or illness that you could make real outcome measures. It is important to realize that the outcome measures being used refer to outcomes of the clinical encounter, not the patient outcomes. One of the issues addressed later on in this chapter is the relative importance of process versus outcome measurements.

Reliability

This is the extent to which the scores achieved by the individual students are truely due to differences in their capabilities, uncontaminated by events or factors over which the examiner has little or no control. Depending on the specific measurement being made, factors such as age, sex, student backgrounds, time, and sequence of tests may influence the behavior measured and lower the reliability of the test tool. Inter-examiner reliability is a common concern in most of the tools used to assess clinical performance. The extent to which two examiners will evaluate the same performance or behavior with the same score(s) will determine the extent to which the measurement made is reliable.

    This consistency of measurement, free of the effect of uncontrolled or confounding variables, is only one aspect of reliability. The second aspect of reliability refers to sampling error. If the test or tool samples a restricted area of skills or knowledge, it may not provide an accurate measurement of the student's overall ability. It may have, by chance, sampled a student's particular area of strength or a particular area of weakness and, therefore, have given an untrue or unreliable estimate of the student's capabilities.

Validity

This refers to the extent to which the test or tool provides an accurate, true reflection of the characteristic it is purported to measure. This is a particular concern in all tests used to measure aspects or characteristics of problem-solving or clinical reasoning skills. Is this what they are really measuring, or are they in fact measuring something else? Face validity is a less rigorous estimate of validity, as it only requires that the teacher, or an expert in the subject area of the test, feels that the test does indeed measure the characteristics in question. It can be said to have face validity if the student, on taking the test, also feels that the test is valid. Content validity indicates that these same people would feel that the content of the test adequately samples the area of information to be measured. Concurrent and construct validity can be more rigorous estimates of validity. The former requires that the result of the tests in question, when compared to the results of other tests that have an established validity, and are taken at the same time, would show a significant correlation. The latter requires that the result of the test in question, when compared against a logical construct or hypothesis about the characteristic tested, will show correlation. For example, it is a reasonable hypothesis that clinical reasoning skills should improve from year to year in medical school and continue to improve during postgraduate training; therefore, a test purported to test clinical reasoning or a subset of clinical reasoning, if given to the student at these levels, should be expected to show increasing scores for students at more advanced levels. Predictive validity is a powerful requirement in validity. It requires the score of the student to bear a strong relationship to his ability to apply the characteristic tested in the real-life, day-to-day, working situation. The ideal test for clinical reasoning at the specialty board or fellowship level is one that has predictive validity.

Fidelity

This attribute is interrelated with validity and describes the extent to which the test resembles or mimics the real-life setting in which the characteristic is to be measured. Performance measured in a real-life environment more accurately reflects the performance that will occur in real life. We can expect that tests using high-fidelity teaching tools, such as the airline's cockpit simulator, computer-driven human mannequins, and simulated patients will offer a greater predictive validity for clinical reasoning skills and patient care skills.

Feasibility

This refers to the logistic difficulties (that are unrelated to the behavior measured) that the student may encounter in taking the test, as well as the ease with which the faculty can provide the test. Factors that affect the feasibility are cost, ease of reproduction, portability, and most important, ease of use. For example, the computer or P4 can be complex to use, as compared to true–false tests, and the computer has the added disadvantage of not generally being portable or available in large numbers. From the faculty standpoint, feasibility also involves the ease with which results can be scored and analyzed. Compare the teacher's job in scoring essay questions with that of true-false questions. Compare the problems of watching and scoring a chain of students doing patient history and physical examination for an entire day, as opposed to scoring the formulation and treatment plans written on a piece of paper.

Reliable Evaluation Tools with Questionable Validity

The first group considered includes examinations with high reliability but a questionable validity in their ability to assess parts of the clinical reasoning process or clinical competence.

Multiple-Choice/True-False Questions

This format has been developed into a very sophisticated method for the assessment of content knowledge in medicine (Hubbard et al., 1965; Newble, 1975; Barro, 1973). Such "objective" examination items have, over the years, developed a well-established reliability. These questions can be presented in a variety of formats, such as the one best response, matching response, evaluation of possibly related phrases, and multiple-choice and true-false questions. In these tests, the student is required only to select or mark the correct option or options. As a result, the student can be challenged with a large number of questions in a short time. This allows the questions to screen or sample from wide areas of content, increasing the reliability of the student's score as an accurate representation of his overall knowledge. All this, combined with the ease and low cost of administering and scoring these questions for any number of students in any location, makes this evaluation tool a most attractive format and, together with its reliability, accounts for its universal popularity.

Considerable skill and science are involved in writing good multiple-choice or true-false questions. The unskilled question writer can easily suggest the right answer to the student by allowing any of a variety of almost unconsciously perceived cues to occur. The amateur writer may obscure the meaning or intent of a question, confusing the student with verbal contortions in his attempt to put a particular point into the question format.

The issue of validity is the major drawback to the use of this format. It seems quite evident from many studies that the basic behavior evaluated is the pure recall of information necessary to make the correct choice. Even in those questions that are cleverly designed to test the student's reasoning by asking him to interpret information and make diagnostic or therapeutic decisions, the correct choice is always in front of him or, as in the case of true-false or phrase-comparing questions, it is merely the choice of right or wrong. The PMP format represents a redesign of this multiple-choice question format so that it more closely resembles the cognitive challenge of the patient problem setting, yet without loss of its inherent reliability. As stated many times earlier, there is no evidence that the pure recall of information, despite the fact that it is well tested, in any way correlates with competence in clinical reasoning or the care of patients; therefore, if multiple-choice, true-false questions are used in student assessment for problem-based learning, it must be with the realization that they provide a reliable method of widely sampling information recall. Their ability to assess other behaviors, including the ability to apply recalled information appropriately in the clinical reasoning process, is problematic or speculative. This format certainly cannot evaluate the student's inquiry strategies, problem formulation skills or any of his clinical or interpersonal skills.

Word-Completion or Short-Answer Questions

Much of what has been said about multiple-choice, true-false questions applies here as well. These questions have the advantage of not cueing the student to the right answer, but provide him with a blank space instead, in which he is to recall it on his own. Although they also have a questionable validity, it is conceivable that they could estimate the student's ability to perceive the importance of data or interpret its meaning. They could evaluate his ability to generate hypotheses on initial cues and make diagnostic or therapeutic decisions on the information presented. With the alternative tools that are available for evaluation, however, the question may not be worth pursuing. These questions test recall best, do not evaluate segments of the clinical reasoning process well, and cannot in any way evaluate inquiry strategies or clinical or interpersonal skills. Scoring has to be done by hand and the criterion for the right answer may not be as clear cut in this format, requiring some interpretation by those who review the answers and permitting a source of bias in scoring.

Evaluation Tools with Poor Reliability and Questionable Validity

The next set of examinations to be considered includes those with a very poor reliability because of the bias introduced by the subjectiveness of the evaluation. These forms of examination also have questionable validity in assessing components in the clinical reasoning process or clinical competence.

Oral Examination

This is another long-standing, traditionally employed method of student assessment. It has the advantage of establishing a dialogue or interaction between the student and the examiner. It gives the examiner the opportunity to sense the student's capabilities in a diagnostic sense and to explore his areas of strength and weakness in terms of knowledge and thinking ability. The oral examination represents a problem-solving process for the examiner: he can ask those questions that relate to the hypotheses that occur in his mind regarding the student's performance, possible areas of ignorance, or poor capabilities. It is, in this sense, a potent tool for probing the student's knowledge and understanding in a variety of areas and for seeing if he can apply the knowledge he has to more advanced concepts or problems presented to him by the examiner. The examiner can determine his ability to interpret symptoms or signs; to formulate a patient's problem; to suggest hypotheses for the problem presented; and to describe decisions in diagnosis and treatment, continuing management, and the like. The examiner also can gain a sense about the student's self-evaluation or self-study approaches by asking him how he feels he has done so far in the curriculum or in the oral examination. He can ask the student about the questions the student feels he needs to pursue as a consequence of the oral examination and what resources he would, or did use in the past. It is even possible for the examiner to use role playing to obtain an idea about the student's skills. This is a technique that has been used in a number of evaluation situations, particularly in the specialty of orthopedics. The oral exam is unlike other evaluation procedures in that the examiner can get a feel for the student's personality and can see how the student may react or reason under pressure or stresses, which the examiner, in his position, can apply easily in the interpersonal examiner–student situation.

Although this is a versatile and flexible tool, it is virtually crippled by the overwhelming problems of reliability and by some problems in validity. The personal biases of the examiner are almost impossible to avoid. His concept of how much a student should know is very personal; he has never had the chance to review it objectively with the other faculty and it is largely based on his own experiences and convictions. Even his biases on how the student should dress and behave, nonverbally and verbally, can affect his overall evaluation. Attempts to standardize or control this assessment for these variables in the encounter require considerable training of examiners. The interpersonal dynamics of the interaction and the artificiality of the verbal presentation of patient data, plus the interpersonal stresses unique to that situation, make its validity open to question. Also, despite the range of competencies that can be tested, it seems that the majority of the evaluations done in this mode are at the content recall level.

This is an excellent, personal evaluation method by which a teacher can probe content knowledge and the ability to communicate verbally, as well as gain some insights about the student's clinical reasoning process and his ability to reason in general. It is a highly unreliable method to use for any objective assessment of capabilities. It is certainly best suited to providing the student with personal feedback about the teacher's concept of his strengths and weaknesses. It is treacherous if used as a method for grading or certifying the student's abilities.

Essay Examination

This is an excellent method for determining how well a student writes or can communicate his thoughts verbally. His ability to organize and express ideas can be evaluated, and some measure of his personal creativity can be obtained. Again, it is a highly unreliable tool because of the difficulty in achieving any precision or objectivity in scoring. Marking is difficult and time consuming. There is good reason to question the validity of assuming that the student's ability to express his ideas and thoughts in writing correlates with his ability to use clinical reasoning with a medical problem.

Valid Evaluation Tools with Questionable Reliability

The next set of evaluation procedures includes those that have face validity (in some instances construct and/or concurrent validity) in their assessment of cognitive skills related to clinical reasoning and clinical competence. The major problem to date has been that a proven ability to develop and rank hypotheses and propose management for a cardiac problem may not be duplicated by the same student when faced with a neurological problem. Measures of process (techniques of interview, examination, and the like) tend to possess greater reliability across problem areas, but their ability to predict the overall quality of performance is questionable.

Observation of a Patient Interview and Examination

The paradoxical aspect of measurement tools is shown best here. The observation of a student interviewing a real (or simulated) patient has obvious validity to the clinical situation. The student is being evaluated while performing his real-world, professional task, yet this type of examination is highly unreliable. The criteria for the student performance are difficult to standardize. Good rating scales do not exist. The ones most conventionally used have difficulty in insuring the application of standardized criteria for each student and in providing for inter-examiner reliability. The biases of each examiner are a problem when criteria to be employed in measurement are not clear cut. There is a perpetual "centralizing" tendency among faculty examiners. Fearing commitment at either the low or unsatisfactory end of a measurement scale or commitment at the high or most competent end, they tend to score students in the middle (2 on a scale of 3, 3 on a scale of 5). This prevents any separation of skills among students or provision of a meaningful measurement. This fear, of course, is engendered partly by the lack of clear-cut, understandable criteria on which the student can be scored.

Another problem, related to the use of patients, is that the patient brings a wide variety of uncontrolled and unknown variables into the encounter. In the usual situation, the faculty who are observing the student rarely have the chance to use a patient whose condition has been known well enough to allow well-defined criteria for the student's performance with that patient. If the patient is known well enough by the faculty, it usually means that this is a patient that has a chronic illness and has been seen many times. Such repeated contact with the physicians and students invariably produces a patient that no longer presents the picture of the naive, concerned layman with an illness. He has been educated by the many questions, examinations, and educations he has received about his illness and, as a consequence, is atypical of the majority of patients the physician eventually will see. In addition, the patient may vary widely in his answers to questions, memory of past events, interpretation of symptoms, and even in his findings. This fact is well known to house staff, who present patients on rounds the day following their evaluation of the patient, only to find the history and findings totally different. Lastly, the patient may have confounding complications, communication difficulties, or be deteriorating clinically, which may hamper the student's performance unfairly, Again, this is not to say that this is not a good method of evaluation, as much information about the student's abilities to perform his most important skills can be obtained, but it will never be an *accurate* assessment that can produce meaningful data about the student, his true capability, and his relationship to other students at his particular educational level.

The student can demonstrate his inquiry skills, his ability to choose appropriate questions and physical examination items, and his ability to interview and examine. His use of time can be evaluated in the clinical situation. It is difficult through observation, however, to learn anything about the student's perception of data from the patient and his interpretation of that data. His problem formulation and hypotheses also are difficult to evaluate. If the student's encounter with a patient is videotaped for subsequent review, then these important elements of the clinical reasoning process can be evaluated better on an individual basis.

The use of the simulated patient can improve the reliability of this assessment procedure by providing a patient problem that cannot be distinguished from real life yet can be known in every detail so that the faculty can determine specific criteria for student performance. The simulated patient is free of unplanned and uncontrollable variables and can present himself as real and fresh to each student. Most important, the problems can be selected far enough in advance so that the faculty can prepare their criteria on the basis of the performances of faculty experts who have worked with the same patient problem. (This will be discussed later.) Since the same problem can be offered to many students, year after year, realistic performance measurements can be made (Barrows, 1971; Burri et al., 1976).

Observing a student working with a patient or simulated patient is used frequently to evaluate interpersonal, physician–patient skills. Again, important estimations can be made, but it is important to realize that the third party viewing the encounter between the student and patient does not really perceive the manner and appearance of the student that the patient perceives. Frequently, patients and simulated patients will report quite different feelings about the student's interpersonal skills, his manner, and his rapport, than will an observer of the interaction. The evaluation of interpersonal skills can be enhanced by using simulated patients who are trained to give the student feedback as to their feelings about the interaction.

In conclusion, the observation of a student–patient encounter allows the teacher to estimate inquiry strategy, history taking, physical examination skills, and use of time, with considerable validity. The low reliability of this tool can be improved by the use of simulated patients and by training observers for scoring. Videotaping the encounter allows the teacher to estimate skills in data interpretation and perception, as well as problem formulation and hypothesis generation, and provides the student with an excellent tool for self-evaluation.

Review of Case Record

A mechanism for using this format for learning and evaluation has been developed by Weed (1969) and others. There are the same reliability concerns as previously expressed in the observation of a patient encounter. Again, this can be improved, if needed, by the use of simulated patients. This tool can evaluate a student's ability to recognize important data coming from the patient problem and to interpret that data. His problem formulation can be evaluated, as can his decisions, diagnoses, and treatment. Some impression can be gained of his ideas or skills in continuing care of the patient problem and of the cost of his evaluation. The case record is easier to score than is direct observation. His generation of hypotheses and inquiry strategy cannot be evaluated well. The case report complements the observation of the student's examination by providing information that cannot be evaluated during the encounter. The patient's report also will evaluate the student's ability to communicate in writing, his organization and expression, and his ability to write patient orders.

If a simulated patient were used in the evaluation, the student would be able to refer subsequently to the write up of experts who have encountered the same simulation, thus exercising his skills in self-evaluation.

The extension of this evaluation tool is the record audit, used more frequently in postgraduate and continuing medical educational settings. The techniques employed to create criteria for the "indicator conditions" selected for review have increased the reliability (Spitzer et al., 1974). The main advantage is that the record audit tells you what the physician or student really did in his work with patients, as opposed to what in single-encounter records they say that they will do. Most of the evaluation tools described assess what the student says that he will do in the treatment and management of patients. This distinct advantage of the record audit makes it an excellent tool for looking at the student's skills, the sequential or continuing care of the patient problem, and its cost. Again, such record audits totally ignore clinical skills and interpersonal skills.

Patient Problem Simulations

The next group of evaluation techniques are based on the simulation of the patient problem. The accuracy with which behaviors evaluated with a patient simulation format reflect those behaviors that would actually be seen in the real-life clinical setting depend largely on the fidelity of the simulation (the extent to which it represents the real world).

Patient Management Problems

This is an increasingly popular printed format, pioneered by McGuire & Babbott (1967), that can be produced in large numbers and scored easily. Experience has been accumulated with its use in a variety of certifying examinations. In this format, an initial amount of patient data is presented to the student, usually more than would be true in the real clinical situation. On the basis of this data the student is then asked to choose, from a list of possibilities, the action he would take. The result of his choice usually is revealed by the use of an invisible ink made visible by felt marker, or by erasing an opaque coating or removing a tab covering the result of the action. The student also is referred to more information as he makes more choices. When he receives the result of his choice, he usually is referred to another section of the problem where further information about the patient is disclosed and new choices need to be made. In this manner, the student is forced to commit himself in terms of data analysis and diagnostic and treatment decisions. He is forced to follow the consequences of his choices with a patient problem. Its greatest asset is in its ease of scoring; however, several studies have indicated that validity is limited in this format (Feightner & Norman, 1976; Goran et al., 1973). The student is cued by the limited choices available, similar to the way he is cued by multiple-choice questions. The student is not free to take whatever action he might like with the patient. He is forced to make choices from a specific category of choices and then is referred to another category of choices for further decision. He is not able to tackle the problem in any sequence, unlike the real situation. As a result, he is unable to employ freely his inquiry strategy, limiting this simulation's similarity to the challenge of the clinical situation. Nevertheless, the student's perception and interpretation of data and, to a limited degree, his inquiry strategy and his diagnostic and treatment decisions can be evaluated. The information that he can recall to apply to the problem can be evaluated, as can his ability to continue on in the care of a patient problem. This is a good tool for the student who wishes to evaluate himself at various points in the problem format against the expert's criteria for decision making.

Sequential Management Problems

This is a relatively new name for an older format that we originally called the "problem box" (Barrows & Mitchell, 1975). In this evaluation format, the student is presented with an initial or opening statement about the patient and the setting in which the patient problem is encountered and is asked to describe what he thinks may be going on in the patient problem and what actions he would take next. His written perception and interpretation of initial data, and possibly the hypotheses he would generate early in the problem, can be evaluated. He can either commit himself in writing or make a choice from options, as in the patient management problem (PMP). (Use of the latter choice raises the same concerns about cueing.) Once the student has committed himself, he then turns to the next section in the sequential management problem, which describes what was actually done with the patient and what was found. The text again stops and the student, on the basis of this new information, again describes what he would do next and how he would put the problem together. This allows for evaluation of his problem formulation and, to a certain degree, his inquiry strategy; that is, the specific questions or sequence of questions he would use in this patient problem.

When it comes to the physical examination, the student is asked to describe what he would look for and what he might expect to find. In this

manner, he can be carried through the requesting and interpretation of laboratory tests, the diagnostic decisions, and the therapeutic decisions, and can
continue on with long-term management of the problem. The student is able
to evaluate his decisions at each step by comparing what he decided to do, or
his interpretation of what is going on in the patient, with what is revealed in
the text of the sequential management problem.

Berner (Berner et al., 1974) is responsible for giving this format the
name of sequential management problem (SMP). She felt that the student's
decisions at many points could be evaluated better, particularly in continuing
management decisions, if he were not permitted the freedom that occurs in
the usual patient management problem. In such a case, if the student had
poor skills in inquiry, he could go down the wrong pathway in his management decisions; thus, his ability to carry out other aspects of diagnostic or
therapeutic decisions could not be evaluated. Berner's "linear" format, where
the student is forced to follow the pathway taken by the clinicians described
in the problem, has an advantage in evaluating specific management skills.

It was, however, our dissatisfaction with the linearity of the problem
box, which inhibited the student from pursuing his own inquiry strategy, that
led to the development of the P4 (Tamblyn & Barrows, 1978). Validity to the
clinical reasoning process has not yet been evaluated for sequential management problems. Scoring is more difficult when multiple-choice is not used.
This format can evaluate the perception and interpretation of data, problem
formulation, generation of hypotheses to some degree, inquiry strategies in
terms of the next step the student will take, and continuing management of
the patient problem. It is a useful tool in self-evaluation.

Computer Simulations

There is a variety of computer simulations that have been developed. Some
represent a patient management problem put into a computer format. The
student is presented with a description of the patient problem and then is
given a set of options to choose from. His choice produces more information
and a set of further choices. This has all the advantages and disadvantages of
the patient management problem. An immediate score, however, can be provided, giving instant feedback to the student.

A number of natural-language computer programs have been developed
that allow the student to make his own choice of actions on history, physical
examination, and requesting laboratory tests, and in any sequence. This more
closely simulates the challenge of a patient problem and allows the student to
demonstrate his inquiry strategy in attempting to sort out or rank the hypotheses in his head. This is probably the first format so far that really allows
the student's inquiry strategy, one of the most important segments of the

clinical reasoning process, to be evaluated (Dickinson et al., 1973; Harless, 1971; Friedman, 1973; Friedman et al., 1977).

Improvements are occurring steadily in the computer simulation. Friedman (1973) has developed a computer program in which changes occur in the patient's condition over time and in which the availability of tests can be simulated in terms of the time it takes for the report to be obtained. His program also can calculate the costs of the student's evaluation of the problem. The computer can be linked to audiovisual presentations so that the patient's appearance, X rays, fundoscopic appearances, blood smears, electrocardiograms, heart sounds, and other data can be observed by the student and presented for his interpretation. In this manner, the student's ability to perceive and interpret data can be evaluated.

The computer simulations developed by Dickinson et al. (1973) at McMaster University have complex, interrelated, physiological parameters programmed around a patient's problem in such areas as cardiovascular, respiratory, renal, and drug intoxication problems. As a student attempts to treat the problem, the various physiological and biochemical changes related to his interventions, drugs, and dosage occur. This, like the change over time mentioned previously, takes full advantage of the computer's ability to both allow the student free choice of action and present complex, multiple interrelated phenomena that change over time. As in the patient management problem, the students are committed to their course of action and end up with an improved, unchanged, worsened, or even dead patient; a far better format in which to blunder than in real life.

There are, however, many problems associated with the use of the computer. The major one is expense. Another is the fact that the student is limited to the location of available terminals and the time that they are free. More recently, Friedman et al. (1977) has developed an electronic voice computer that can give patient information over the telephone, eliminating to a large extent the availability problem. The student or physician interacts with a computer through the telephone dial or buttons. A third problem with computer simulations is that interaction with the computer is usually with a keyboard and the use of some variety of code system, even in the natural-language mode. Validity with the computer format has not been evaluated rigorously; some recent studies suggest that it may be low (Feightner & Norman, 1976).

In summary, the computer challenges the student's data perception and interpretation, allows free use of inquiry strategy, and can challenge the ability to intervene with a patient problem in which there are spontaneous changes over time or changes that relate to the treatment that the student has given the patient. The computer can calculate the cost of the patient management and can provide the student with immediate feedback as to score and its relationship to the score of experts or others in his particular peer group. This is a growing and potent format in the evaluation of the clinical reasoning process.

Portable Patient Problem Pack (P4)

The P4 has been mentioned previously and will be described more thoroughly later. It represents a patient problem in a playing-card format, in which the student is given the opening picture and the setting of the patient's problem very much as it would occur in actual life. Subsequently, the student is free to choose any actions in any sequence he wishes. He can ask questions of any variety on interview; perform a variety of physical examination items, laboratory tests, or diagnostic procedures; obtain the opinion of a variety of consultants; and treat the patient with medication, surgery, psychotherapy, hospitalization, or the like. After he has selected an action (card), he can receive the information produced by that action by reading the back of the card. The sequence of cards selected documents his inquiry path, since he has free choice in employing his inquiry strategies (Barrows & Tamblyn, 1977). As this format was designed on the basis of the understanding we now have of the physician's clinical reasoning process, described in Chapter 2, there are design features deliberately built into the format that help the student develop this skill. Audiovisual materials, such as patient photographs, X rays, fundoscopic appearances, and electrocardiograms, are integrated into the pack to challenge the student's ability to observe and interpret these laboratory data.

A variety of evaluation approaches are incorporated into the format. The various cards, or actions the student selects in dealing with the problem, all have been given a value, on a 2+ to a 2− scale, by a panel of experts. When the student has finished working with the problem, he can review his inquiry strategy, looking for blind alleys or inappropriate choices. He can look at the values assigned to the cards and calculate his efficiency and proficiency on the basis of a formula similar to that employed in the PMP. He is given reference material, P4 sequences chosen by experts who have worked with the problem, and patient write ups done by a variety of experts, to assist him in evaluating his own clinical reasoning. To aid him in developing or evaluating areas of self-study, there is a list of appropriate study issues compiled by experts who have reviewed the problem from their particular disciplines (such as anatomy, physiology, rehabilitation, biochemistry, or clinical medicine) and have indicated the appropriate learning issues they feel this problem would stimulate.

Recent work done with the P4, comparing student's behavior working with the P4 to their behavior with the same problem presented by a simulated patient, would suggest that the validity of this format to the clinical situation is quite high (Tamblyn & Barrows, 1978). The ability of this tool to assess a wide range of phenomena in the area of cognitive process, data perception and interpretation, hypothesis generation, problem formulation, inquiry strategy, and diagnostic and therapeutic decision making makes it a particularly valuable tool for evaluation. Since the cards also incorporate a sequential management problem system that allows the student to continue to work with the problem over time, data can be generated that allow continuing management to be evaluated. Evaluation of P4 play, before and after self-study, provides a means of determining the effectiveness of individual student's study skills.

Simulated Patients

The simulated patient already has been discussed in the previous chapters. It represents a normal person carefully trained to simulate accurately a patient problem that has existed or exists at the present time. The simulated patient can escape detection by skilled clinicians, presents a constant problem from student to student, and is an evaluation tool that can be scheduled for a particular time and place in the future, allowing the faculty to decide upon criteria for student performance with a standardized problem. As a consequence, the reliability of the faculty scoring of the clinical interaction can be improved. The reliability of the simulated patient presenting unchanging findings from student to student has been well established in a variety of studies. Its validity can be inferred from the fact that a simulated patient was undetected in actual medical practice situations, on several occasions. The experienced clinicians who worked with the simulated patient believed they were dealing with a real patient and were unaware that it was a simulation.

Since the clinical encounter with the simulated patient can be stopped at any point, faculty have the opportunity to analyze and shape all aspects of the student's clinical reasoning process; in addition, it provides realistic data by which the student's clinical skills (history taking and physical examination) can be evaluated. This is a particularly potent tool for evaluating interpersonal skills, since the simulated patient can be trained to provide accurate feedback to the student from the patient's point of view. Simulated patient feedback has been the aspect of this format that students have found most attractive; it has been mainly their support that has allowed this technique to survive over the last 10 to 15 years.

As a consequence, the simulated patient provides us with an evaluation tool that can look at the whole taxonomy of performances important in patient care and the objectives we feel are important in medical education. If a student is asked to write up a case history following his interaction with the simulated patient, and if the interaction is also videotaped, the faculty then have a complete evaluation tool.

Some of the disadvantages of the simulated patient relate to faculty misunderstanding about the technique. Many faculty have the idea that simulated patients are too artificial to use with students, but, as mentioned before, experience has shown time again that simulated patients have to be seen and experienced before they can be believed. This is a principal problem in encouraging faculty to use this format in teaching and evaluation; however, even the staunchest critics become convinced and enthusiastic about the simulated patient when they have had a face-to-face experience. Students who are told ahead of time that the patient is simulated testify that they soon forget this fact and become engrossed in what seems to be a totally real patient. The same experience is shared by residents, clinicians, and medical faculty. Unfortunately, the term simulated patient has been used as a label for role players, subjects for the physical examination, "pseudo" patients, and a variety of poorly trained simulated patients. All of these rather spurious forms of simulation have given the technique a negative audience in many quarters. Properly trained simulated patients are indistinguishable from real patients and yet provide educational advantages beyond those possible with real patients.

Another concern is that the simulated patient only presents typical or classical disease entities, not the kinds of vague or complex problems without characteristic history or findings that are encountered by the student in the real world. Simulated patients, however, are not "created" from a textbook or a teacher's mind, but are carefully trained to portray an actual patient. All the faculty needs to do is to pick the actual patient problem, diagnosed or undiagnosed, clear or confused, that they want to use to challenge the student's clinical skills.

A third complaint is that it is impossible to simulate many physical signs, such as heart sounds, chest sounds, swollen joints, and edema; therefore, the range of problems that can be simulated is small. This is true, in part, but a sufficient variety of conditions can be simulated to challenge effectively the candidate's clinical skills. The many physical signs that can be simulated include pneumothorax, rales, asthma, dilated pupils, nuchal rigidity, rigid abdomen or guarding, muscle spasm, contractures, joint abnormalities, paralysis, reflex changes, sensory losses, and thyroid bruit. The range extends as creative faculty further explore the use of the tool. Despite this, there is a wide variety of conditions where a careful or probing physical examination is needed to assess the patient, although there are actually no physical signs. Lastly, a whole range of manufactured simulators of sounds, sights, and body lumps and bumps is available to augment the simulated patient. Real patients with fixed findings can be used, either for practice in

the evaluation and interpretation of specific findings or for a different problem that uses the findings they presently have.

It has been felt by many that good, simulated patients are difficult and
time-consuming to prepare. Once the technique for appropriate training has
been learned, it takes only three one-hour sessions to train a person who has
never been a simulated patient. After the simulator has learned his first patient role, it takes one hour or less to prepare him for additional patient
simulations.

Many have felt the simulated patient is too expensive and impractical to
be used in the assessment of hundreds of students at the same time. This may
be a real concern, but not in terms of practicality. Almost any number of
simulated patients can be trained to present the same patient problem with
very little increase in effort. Cost certainly needs to be considered. One simulator can be used to assess approximately ten students if you allow each student up to thirty minutes to evaluate a patient. If one simulated patient is
paid, for example, $100 for a day's work, then each patient simulation costs
$10 per student. To predict any student's abilities, you would probably need
to see him evaluate at least three or four patients presenting a variety of problems, depending upon the evaluation setting and the educational goals. With
the other procedures necessary to complement the use of simulated patients
in an examination situation, the cost may be as much as $50 a student;
however, if you subtract from this the cost of more conventional, less valid or
reliable tests, the simulated patient may not be that expensive. Should we be
concerned if computers, simulated patients, and other techniques are more
expensive? Can a price tag be put on the value of such assessments in terms
of our accountability to the public and responsibility toward the student? If
the assessment techniques used are going to cost the school, the student, or
society any money at all, shouldn't they be as accurate and reliable as possible? The aircraft simulators in the many airports around the world cost
millions of dollars each, and are in constant use in assessing competence because our lives depend on this. The analogy seems obvious.

Mechanical Mannequins

These are mechanical simulations of the human body or portions of the
human body that present a variety of physical signs for the student to observe
and evaluate. The pioneering efforts of Denson & Abrahamson (1969) need
to be acknowledged in this regard. Their production of a model known as
"SIM 1" began as an electronically activated, lifelike, computer-controlled
mannequin used in the training of anesthesiology residents for intratracheal
intubation and anesthetic induction. This very realistic, lifesize dummy
simulates a patient on the operating table. The dummy breathes, has heart

sounds, changes pupillary size, and can receive the laryngoscope and intra-tracheal tube in a very realistic manner. The face can be masked and the arm veins can receive intravenous medication. The pulse can be palpated through the wrist. There is an extensive computer program that both automates the computer and records the various actions the student or resident is taking in the work with the patient. The automation by computer allows the simulation to develop cardiac irregularity, muscle fasciculations, bucking and vomiting, and dilation or constriction of the pupils, all appropriate to the levels of anesthesia, oxygen, and administered drugs. This model can even have its teeth damaged through faulty technique. This is an excellent way for a complex medical skill to be learned at no risk to patients. At the end of the exercise, the computer can give a print-out of the entire performance, detailing time, dose, and many other steps. Dr. Abrahamson has noted recently that this simulated mannequin is capable of training a variety of health professionals, including ward personnel, in a number of approaches to the unresponsive patient (Abrahamson, 1978).

Michael Gordon (1974) at the University of Miami has evolved, over the last few years, a simulated or mechanical mannequin that can present the constellation of findings seen with almost every variety of cardiac disease. As with SIM 1, this allows for repetitive training of students in observing and interpreting physical signs. Because the simulation is under complete control of the faculty, complications can be specified. Most important, the criteria of a competent or acceptable student performance can be specified ahead of time. This is an excellent technique for self-evaluation.

In conclusion, the mechanical mannequins, like the cockpit simulator in aviation, allow the student to both learn and be assessed in the execution of complex skills in observation, physical examination, and medical intervention.

Models

There is a variety of plastic, plaster, metal, and wood dummies that represent mock ups of the various parts of the body and allow the student to be evaluated in his interventions or manipulations. These include models that can be intubated; models in which intravenous therapy can be given; models for the pelvic examination; models for the performance of the lumbar puncture; and models for eye, ear, nose, and throat examination. The range of these models is extensive, increases every year, and offers an important role in the evaluation of motor skills.

Audiovisual Simulation

There is a variety of ways in which audiovisual media can present the student with patient phenomena. Photographs and slides can demonstrate observable findings on the surface of the patient or within the patient's body, as well as morphology, fundoscopic examination, and appearances to various examination apparatus (gastroscopes, sigmoidoscopes). Audiotapes can present cardiac sounds, rales, and gastrointestinal sounds. All of these can present the student with data; the challenge is for him to observe it correctly and interpret its significance. The same audiovisual techniques, of course, can present X rays and a variety of other diagnostic tests.

Videotapes and films can present the total picture of the patient to the student and are particularly valuable for portraying movement or a variety of complex maneuvers. Oftentimes, the videotape or film presentation is used in place of a clinical skills examination such as the interaction with a real patient or a simulated patient. Faculty frequently forget that in doing this they may be challenging the student's ability to make observations and interpret data, but they have sacrificed a great deal of important behavior in the assessment of clinical competence. There is no need to develop interpersonal skills with a videotape or film. There is no opportunity to demonstrate inquiry strategy, the sequence of questions, or the physical examination items that would be done to sort out the hypotheses that are in the student's mind. There is no opportunity to demonstrate ability to interview or perform a physical examination. The videotape or film presentation is not a valid substitute for observation of the student working with a real patient, working with a simulated patient, or even working with a simulation format such as the computer or P4 simulations. In addition, no matter how excellent the videotape or film is, it does not put across the "gestalt" of the patient as effectively as a real patient or a simulated patient.

The only statistical concern in audiovisual evaluation is the manner in which the student responds to what he sees or hears. If he is presented a photograph, slide, or audiotape and then has to score his findings in a multiple-choice format, the usual concerns for validity develop although the reliability may be quite high. If he verbalizes what he sees or writes an essay about his findings, then, of course, inter-examiner reliability and appropriate criteria for scoring can become a concern.

What Should Be Evaluated?

The next step is to identify as closely as possible the individual behaviors or competencies that need to be measured in problem-based learning. Once they have been identified, the evaluation tool can be selected that is suited best to those particular competencies. The following are competencies we need to evaluate in clinical reasoning and problem-based learning.

Clinical Reasoning Skills

Data Perception and Interpretation.   This includes the perception of relevant information from the patient and the problem setting, such as visual, auditory, tactile, verbal, and nonverbal information. Perceptions and interpretations of data from X rays, diagnostic tests, and other written materials provide further information about the patient and his problems. Data interpretation refers to the meaning or significance the student gives the data and the way in which he modifies or translates it in his work with a problem. Although this might be considered separately, it is hard to separate from perception in most evaluation approaches. This behavior does not refer to the subsequent assignment of significance or weight to the data perceived, in the student's attempt to sort out his hypotheses. This more analytical or synthetic activity is looked at or evaluated in the next two behaviors.

Problem Formulation.   This refers to the developing picture of the patient in the student's mind. It begins with the initial patient concept he forms from initial cues picked up at the very beginning of the encounter. The problem formulation continues to grow and evolve as more information is obtained during the inquiry process. It should represent a concise and inclusive summary of all the significant positive and negative information obtained from or about the patient. Significance is measured against the hypothesis tool described next. (As in all of these behaviors, the reader may wish to review Chapter 2, where more characteristics of each segment of the clinical reasoning process are considered in more detail.)

Hypothesis Generation.   This is the student's ability to create hypotheses, at the early phase of the encounter, that will catch all the possible data. It refers not only to the early generation of multiple hypotheses but also to their appropriateness, in terms of specificity, range, and number, to the patient problem as it unfolds. It also refers to the student's ability to rank, modify, eliminate, or verify these hypotheses on the basis of the data obtained. Both clinical hypotheses or hypotheses about basic mechanisms responsible for the problem, as well as hypotheses concerning possible management or treatment programs, may be appropriate for a particular problem, depending upon the educational objectives and the problem itself.

Inquiry Strategy.   This term encompasses the type and sequence of actions taken by the student to help eliminate, verify, or rank the hypotheses. A strategy may include actions on history, physical examination, investigations, or treatment. The reasoning used by the student for using actions relevant to his hypotheses, actions that employ appropriate heuristics in the search for significant data, can be evaluated. Inquiry strategy also refers to the student's ability to scan for background data or new cues when his hypothesis-oriented search becomes unproductive. Techniques used to establish effective communication or rapport can be considered as part of his overall strategy of inquiry into the patient's problem.

Diagnostic Decisions. Decision making is a crucial aspect of the student's skills. He always will have to make diagnostic and management decisions at the appropriate time in the encounter with a patient. When is the evidence sufficient to make a diagnostic decision? How specific should the diagnosis be? Should there be a differential diagnostic list or problem list? The student's skill in making such decisions on the basis of usually insufficient or conflicting information is important to evaluate. The term diagnostic list is not used to imply that a formal or specific diagnosis is necessary. It refers to whatever evaluative decisions have been made during the inquiry on the basis of hypotheses. This can be a simple problem statement, a series of unproved impressions, or a refined diagnosis, as appropriate.

Therapeutic Decisions. This refers to the decisions on which the whole clinical reasoning process is predicated. It represents the deployment of the physician's skill in the care of his patient. The prior diagnostic decisions are a vehicle for this decision, revealing the target at which the therapy is to be aimed. Again, decisions may have to be made on insufficient or conflicting data. These decisions must consider payoff, risk to the patient, cost, possible compliance, and evidence of treatment effectiveness. On occasion, in complex or urgent conditions, these decisions may have to be made before diagnostic decisions are possible or completed.

Time. The previous six behaviors look at the effectiveness of the student's clinical reasoning skills. This one, as well as the next, looks at the efficiency. How long does the student take to evaluate and treat the patient?

Cost. What are the costs of the student's investigations, tests, use of equipment, facilities, consultants, and other health personnel? Though these last two evaluations often are not performed, economy represents an increasingly important aspect of the student's education because the cost of health-care delivery is an increasing national and international concern. Costs can be minimized in large part through skill and efficiency employed by the physician in avoiding redundant tests, unnecessary procedures, and unnecessary use of personnel or facilities.

Sequential Management. This looks at the student's ability to provide continuing care to the patient, to re-evaluate the problem, to sense complications or new directions, and to provide for the patient's medical, educational, and psychosocial needs.

Information Acquired. The effectiveness and efficiency of the clinical reasoning process are affected by the prior knowledge and skills possessed by the student. In many situations, both students and teachers would like to assess the knowledge base that the student brings to his work with the problem or that he has acquired after his self-directed study with a problem. This, then, is an evaluation of his ability to recall facts, concepts, and principles, in a variety of areas that are relevant to the problem study.

Clinical (Technical) Skills

This includes performance of psychomotor skills required of the student in almost any clinical situation. They may need to be expanded for students in different health settings and in more specialized clinical or postgraduate areas. *Interview* and *physical examination* skills are extremely important; in addition, evaluation must touch on the following.

Skills in the Performance of Diagnostic and Therapeutic Procedures. This includes the performance of a lumbar puncture, vena puncture, suturing, and techniques such as electrocardiography or others that may be considered appropriate by the faculty.

Prescription and Order-Writing Skills. This may not be considered necessary, but it includes the clarity and precision with which the student writes orders for others, such as pharmacists and nurses. This might be considered a component of communication skills.

Interpersonal Skills. This refers to the student's ability to establish rapport and communication with the patient, the parents, or other members of the patient's family involved in the situation. It may include his ability to educate the patient about his problem, his role in managing it, and the type of therapy or management program to be initiated. His ability to develop a working relationship with other health professionals also may be of concern.

Communication Skills. This evaluates the student's ability to present information, including case histories, research findings, or his point of view, in either spoken or written form.

Self-Study Skills

Self-Evaluation. This refers to the student's ability to utilize real or simulated-patient experiences to assess his strength and weaknesses in clinical reasoning, interview, examination, interpersonal skills, and the knowledge he brings to bear on the problem.

Study-Question Design. This evaluates the student's ability to pull together his own personal goals, the school and course goals, and the particular needs that have arisen in his work with the problem, into an ordered series of focused questions appropriate for a relevant study plan.

Use of Resources. This refers to the student's ability to use effectively reference books, the library, computer searches, and audiovisual equipment. It often requires an ability to communicate his educational needs to peers, faculty, or experts.

New Information. It is important in many instances to try and determine the scope, depth, and accuracy of information acquired by the student in self-directed study, to be certain that his learning has helped him to gain the kinds of information he needs to work effectively with the problem at hand, as well as meet the objectives of the course or the school.

Summary

This is a basic list of behaviors and capabilities that need to be assessed to ensure that students attain the overall objectives felt to be important for medical students, as well as the skills necessary for problem-based learning. It is neither definitive nor complete.

One behavior that has not been included is student attitude. As important as it is, attitude assessment is a most difficult area and most tools are limited to either personality inventories or structured observation by teachers or other health personnel who work with the student. This latter assessment can be in anecdotal, personal opinion, or structured assessment form. The student's attitudes about people, their needs, their sensitivities and rights, the responsibilities of a physician as a professional, and the motivation that led to medicine all affect the quality of care that a student will give as a physician. Will the student get up in the middle of the night and see the patient when he is a physician? Will he be motivated to cope with a difficult spouse or family of the patient, by communicating with them and attempting to understand their needs? Many difficult issues are involved in any assessment of this important aspect of behavior. Further, it has been questioned whether any effective change in basic attitudes can be accomplished with students of adult age who have completed many years of college. This raises the issue as to whether such evaluations of attitude, if used, should not be used in the selection of applicants for medical school.

Matching Tools to Needs

The following is a review of the efficiency of specific evaluation tools for assessing the behaviors discussed in the previous section (See Table 7-1).

Oral Examination and Essay Test

These are excellent tools for giving the teacher a "feel" for the extent and quality of the student's knowledge and his ability to reason, analyze, synthesize, and express himself. It has diagnostic value for the teacher, since it can sense difficulties present in the student. In addition, the student can learn, from the problems he had during the exam, where he is weak in either his knowledge base, his clarity of thinking, or his ability to express himself. Unfortunately, these examinations tend to degenerate into explorations of content information. At best, they are uncontrolled happenings that are open to personal bias. What intellectual or cognitive processes are demonstrated, although of considerable importance, may not be valid to the processes required in clinical reasoning.

Objective Evaluation, Multiple-Choice, and True–False Tests

These can survey broadly the student's ability to recall information, concepts, and principles from many areas of knowledge. They are convenient, common, and can be reliable. No matter how they are used or designed, they cannot test problem solving. Even if they could, it is doubtful whether the aspects they could test would be valid to the problem solving processes used in clinical reasoning. They should be employed to test content knowledge only.

Observation of Patient Work-Up, Oral Presentation of Patient Problem, or Review of Write-Up

These can provide valid data about many aspects of the clinical reasoning process and clinical, technical, and communication skills. A videotape review of the student's encounter provides the opportunity to interview him about

Table 7-1. This shows the relationship of various evaluation formats to patient-assessment and patient-care skills. The left margin lists a wide variety of possible evaluation formats and tools described in the text. The upper margin lists individual components of the clinical reasoning process, as well as other behaviors identified as being important in the physician's performance, all of which can be evaluated. The legend describes the degree of usefulness of each evaluation tool in measuring each particular behavior.

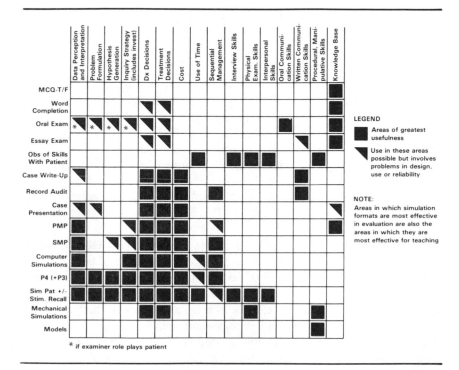

LEGEND

■ Areas of greatest usefulness

◣ Use in these areas possible but involves problems in design, use or reliability

NOTE:
Areas in which simulation formats are most effective in evaluation are also the areas in which they are most effective for teaching

* if examiner role plays patient

his thinking skills, problem formulation, hypothesis generation, and details of diagnostic and therapeutic decision making, as well as the student's background knowledge appropriate to the problem. Assessment of these behaviors in this manner can be improved by standardized interview probes that reduce the inherent problem of observer bias.

The use of actual patients is valuable and evaluates the student's ability to handle a variety of problems with a wide range of findings and complications, both medical and psychosocial; however, it prevents comparative measurements with peers or experts. The competencies expected in both process and outcome can not be precise and the problems best suited for evaluation can not be prescribed ahead of time.

The use of simulated patients allows for more precise and comparative evaluation to occur and for the selection of the problems appropriate for use in the particular evaluation, including the complex and urgent problems generally unavailable for student evaluation. If simulated patients are properly trained and utilized, nothing offered by the real patient is sacrificed.

The examiner represents a source of observer bias in the evaluation setting. An evaluation design should attend to this problem by ensuring that criteria for performance have been specified clearly, scoring is well understood, and examiners are appropriately trained and pretested.

Record Audits

These may provide accurate and reliable information on therapeutic decisions, sequential management, cost, and written communication skills. They seem very limited in assessing any other competency or skill in clinical reasoning or in clinical or technical skills. Their main advantage is that they do show what the student actually did, as opposed to what he says he will do. This format can give some idea about true outcome measures in patient care.

Simulations of Patient Problems

These are amenable to standardization and so they enhance reliability and the possible predictive validity of the evaluation instruments. They place the student in a situation that attempts to mimic accurately some of the important cognitive and psychomotor challenges presented by the real patient. In doing this, sacrifices have to be made in some aspects of fidelity to the real patient problem, in order to achieve important gains in measurement. For example, the PMP, the P4, and computer simulations sacrifice the appearance, sound, and feel of the patient for gains in reproduceability, portability, reliability, ability to evaluate cost of care, and ease and accuracy of measurement. The PMP gains in reliability, low cost, and reproduceability, but loses in the freedom of inquiry strategy and in possible validity. Computer simulations are costly and the problems of maintenance, the numbers and locations of terminals, and the manner of interaction with the computer are a concern in both use and validity. Computers, however, can make the patient problem, as well as the results of investigation, change over time and can provide immediate printout feedback to the student. The P4 allows all of the segments of the clinical reasoning process to be evaluated. It is a very flexible tool for a wide range of evaluations and may have concurrent validity. It is complex to design, although easily reproduced and low in cost. None of these formats can examine clinical, technical, or interpersonal skills.

Simulated Patient

This has the advantage of being an exact substitute, in all respects, for a real patient; yet the simulated patient can be adapted easily to a wide variety of evaluative techniques that permit the complete assessment of clinical reasoning skills, clinical skills, and, particularly, interpersonal skills. Most of the assumed drawbacks to this evaluation tool are fictitious. Cost is moderate. The training and use of simulated patients, although not difficult or time-consuming, has to be learned. Assessment of technical skills concerning treatment and diagnostic interventions are not possible with this variety of simulation.

Models and Mechanical Simulations

These allow the student's skills of observation, examination, and manipulation to be evaluated through simulations that present selected aspects of the patient's appearance, feel, sounds, or responsiveness. They allow the student to be evaluated in performing what could be hazardous techniques if done on real or simulated patients. They also allow for student comparison and the construction of precise criteria of performance, since the problem simulated can be repeated without variation.

Other Possibilities

The evaluator can orchestrate these tools to simulate the total challenge of the real patient for the purposes of an evaluation exercise. For example, after working with a simulated patient where interview, examination, and interpersonal skills are evaluated, the student can take the data he has acquired and write up the case for further analysis. Subsequently, he can be presented with the X ray that he requested, or other test results (usually obtained from the actual patient on which the simulation was based), and his ability to interpret the results and apply them to a reassessment or new approach to the problem can be evaluated. He could return to the simulated patient, who has been programmed to show changes that have occurred in the patient problem, whenever the next encounter is designed to occur in the evaluation: an hour, a day, a week, a month, or a year later.

    An alternate method of assessing ongoing evaluation and management, following the initial simulated patient encounter, would be to give the student access to a computer terminal or P4 simulating the same problem. These would continue to evaluate his choice of investigations or tests, use of consultants, treatment decisions, and ability to carry out his sequential management of the problem without faculty attendance.

If there are certain manipulations that should be evaluated in the student's care of the problem, he could be presented with a model or mechanical simulation. For example, during the examination of a simulated patient in coma, the student may decide that intubation or a lumbar puncture is appropriate; he could demonstrate his skills on the appropriate model.

The disadvantage to mechanical P4, PMP, or computer simulations is that they cannot be interviewed. If interview and interpersonal skills are an important aspect of the evaluation, an interview with a simulated patient, who presents the same problem, can precede work with these other formats.

In all of these simulations, the multiple-choice or true-false test might be integrated into the evaluation, in order to survey the information the student brings to the problem.

Multiple Techniques in Evaluation

Evaluation techniques can be as creative as the teaching techniques in problem-based learning. The only requirements are that the teacher knows what he wishes to accomplish, what his objectives are, and what the tools he is using can and cannot accomplish. Several multiple-assessment approaches have been employed in this manner.

Objective Clinical Examination

Harden (1975) at the University of Dundee, has evloved an "objective clinical examination" that provides a range of evaluations for students. To provide evaluation for students in their clinical terms, he sets up eighteen stations. In two of the stations, the student is required to take a brief history in a specified area from the simulated patient. At the station following each of these stations where there is a simulated patient, the student has to answer objective questions concerning the information he has obtained. At another station the student has to inspect a colored transparency and at the following station answer multiple-choice questions concerning his observations. At five stations, the technique of examination is observed and scored, as performed on normal subjects who provide information concerning the student's technique. These examinations are in specific areas of the body, such as the abdomen or the lower extremities. In this manner, Harden is able to set up an examination procedure that can be reproduced in a number of locations and can survey, in a fairly objective and reliable manner, a wide range of student skills in the clinical setting.

Self-Assessment Units

These were designed to accomplish four objectives. The first was to obviate the need for faculty to spend the time necessary for continuous direct observation of a clinical encounter with a real or simulated patient. The second was to provide an evaluation tool that would examine all aspects of the student's clinical reasoning skills. The third was to provide an evaluation tool that could be used by the student alone for his self-assessment, giving him accurate information about his progress and encouraging skills in continued self-evaluation. Fourth, it was designed to be useful for faculty who wish to use the assessment tool for their own formative or summative evaluation of students.

The operation of this unit requires only a simulated patient, an appropriate room for a clinical examination, and a videotape machine. The student turns on the television apparatus that records the clinical encounter. He then interviews and examines a simulated patient for a specified length of time, usually 30 minutes. When the simulated patient encounter is ended, the student moves to a desk in a quiet room where there is a pile of papers; he is asked to take each in order. The first paper on the stack is a blank sheet of paper for him to write up his patient problem, using the format desired in the educational program; for example, a problem-oriented write-up or the usual case write-up. If the student is at an earlier level in his learning, perhaps recording his data base, his synthesis of the problem, his understanding of the basic mechanisms, and some idea of how he might treat would be appropriate. The next items on the stack are a series of multiple-choice, true–false questions that are addressed to a wide range of issues in basic science and clinical medicine and are related to that patient problem. Once he has answered those questions, he uses the next sheet on the stack, an answer sheet, to score himself and see in what areas he made mistakes or had incorrect information, where further study might be profitable. At the same time, he also learns where he has adequate or in-depth knowledge. As this process is going on, the student becomes more distant from his clinical encounter and more sophisticated. The next item on the stack of sheets is a problem-oriented assessment and management plan, written by an expert physician who had examined previously the same simulated patient, as an unknown. The student is asked to compare this formulation with his own and he is asked to critique both of them. When this is completed, he moves to a videotape playback unit where a videotape can be seen of this expert physician's interview and examination of the same simulated patient. The student is asked to note any items in the expert's evaluation of the patient that he thinks might be valuable to learn. His prior review of the expert's problem-oriented record should cue him for areas where his own assessment may be inadequate or different from that of the expert. The student then receives a report, filled out by the simulated patient, on the student's interpersonal skills. This is a structured report and contains the simulated patient's reaction to the student's approach and manner. The student is asked to note these observations, say whether or not he agrees with them, and indicate what items in his own performance he might like to review as a consequence.

At this point, considerable time has elapsed since the original examination of the simulated patient, so the student may be more objective about seeing his own performance replayed; at the same time, he has gained considerable knowledge, from the various items he reviewed, about the kind of problem the patient presents. He now is prepared for an objective evaluation of his own performance. Given an evaluation form for the clinical performance of medical students, he sits down and evaluates his interview and examination of the patient. At the completion of this session, the student has a variety of evaluative materials through which he can survey his ability to deal with that patient problem, his cognitive skills, his clinical or technical skills, his knowledge base, and his interpersonal skills. He now has the option of sitting down with a faculty member and reviewing areas of concern and question.

It is quite clear that such units also can be used by faculty to assess a student's performance at many levels. Experience has shown that these units are quite motivating for the students because they are able to achieve substantial insights about their strengths and weaknesses. They also have been used as tools to assess carefully the clinical skills of students the faculty may feel are insecure in some aspect of their clinical reasoning or their work with patients. In these instances, it is used as a diagnostic tool (Barrows & Tamblyn, 1977).

Paired or Matched Problems

One valuable and often neglected method for evaluation is the use of the paired problem. When the student or students have completed work with the patient problem in a particular format, they can take on a similar or matched problem to see if they are more efficient or effective in their work with that problem. They can see if the approaches in clinical reasoning or the knowledge acquired can be employed effectively and result in improved skills. A matched problem is not always easy to find or develop, since no two problems are exactly alike. It can, however, be matched for the particular objectives that existed when the initial problem was undertaken. For example, if the students worked with a patient problem that featured transverse myelitis and a blind eye (a case of multiple sclerosis) and their objectives were to be able to evaluate the patient problem well enough to locate the lesion or lesions involved and to understand the anatomical pathways, another problem such as a subacute combined degeneration of the spinal cord might present exactly the same challenges in terms of evaluation, location of lesion, and application of anatomical principles from the same area.

Videotape Recall

This is a particularly valuable technique for evaluating the clinical reasoning process of students at almost any level of medical education. In Chapter 2, this was described as the technique used in a number of studies carried out to analyze the components of the clinician's clinical reasoning process.

During the encounter between the student and the patient or simulated patient, the videocamera should be as unobtrusive as possible. The best arrangement is to record the encounter through one-way glass. The camera should be situated so that the student's face can be seen clearly on the videotape playback. The most potent effect of this recall ("stimulated recall") is its ability to allow the student to relive the episode.

This technique works best if the examiner is relatively nonthreatening for the student. For example, if the patient he examined had cardiological problems, it might be advisable for the faculty who interviews the student to be a family physician or a neurologist, rather than someone who could be perceived as being critical of the student's cardiological ability or knowledge. Carrying this a bit further, it seems quite possible that, with appropriate training, nonphysicians could examine the stimulated recall. In our hands, it has worked quite well with nurses and other people in education. The only important background is their understanding of the clinical reasoning process.

The second important factor in this interview is that the examiner, besides being nonthreatening, be nondirective. This retrospective recall of thinking can be influenced easily by the comments of the examiner. For example, the examiner could ask the student what hypotheses he had in his head shortly after the interaction began. If the student had no hypotheses in his head, or only had one, he might be subtly influenced to come up with hypotheses that really had not occurred to him in the interview. Therefore, the questions should be as open ended as possible. The following questions are suggested for the repertoire of the examiner.

1. "What was going on in your mind at that point?"
2. "Why did you ask that question (or make that comment, or perform that item of examination)?"
3. "What was the patient's problem as you saw it at that point?"
4. Once the student has volunteered that he had some diagnostic ideas

or hypotheses in his mind, the interviewer can ask such questions as, "How did you rank the likelihood of _____ (listing the hypotheses mentioned) at this time?"

Before the videotape recall begins, it is important to orient students to the procedure. The following comments would be helpful.

We would like to know exactly what was going on in your mind as you worked with your patient. Please express any thoughts you had about the nature of the patient's problem, the significance of any symptoms or observations, the reasons for particular questions you asked or things that you did on examination, and concerns you may have had about management and treatment of the patient's problem(s). In addition, please mention any concerns you have about the patient in general, this setting, the simulation (if a simulated patient was used), the room, or any other factors you think are important.

Please don't let the information you now have about the patient influence your comments about what you were thinking at the beginning of your encounter, as you see yourself on the screen. We want to know exactly what was going on in your mind at that time.

Please do not assume that we have any set expectations as to what should have been going on in your mind. Do not formalize or express thoughts or ideas that did not actually occur at the time. In order for this evaluation to be successful, you must attempt to relive your thought processes as accurately as possible.

I will stop the videotape recording at any point at which it occurs to either you or myself that it may be valuable for discussion about thoughts and ideas. Please let me know if this is perfectly clear or if you have any questions.

This is the setup for the videotape recall. Both the interviewer and the student should be comfortably positioned in front of the videotape playback unit and monitor, easily within an arm's distance of the stop or hold switch so that conversation can go on without the videotape progressing. It is important for this recall to occur as shortly after the student's encounter with the patient or simulated patient as possible so that the events that occurred are fresh in the student's mind.

Once the videotape of the encounter has begun, the interviewer should interrupt repeatedly with the kinds of questions just mentioned. It certainly is important to ask, within a few moments of the initial encounter, about what might be going on in the student's mind. Students, physicians, and others who are subjected to this videotape review frequently will deny that they have any ideas or formulations in their minds. To that nondirective question they will answer, "Oh, nothing in particular; I was just asking my usual questions." Whenever they ask questions that seem to be particularly focused toward a diagnosis or hypothesis, however, it is important to ask, "Why did you ask that question (or questions)?" Oftentimes they will reveal a number of hypotheses they have had in their heads all along, yet had not mentioned in the beginning. It is important for you to ask them then to estimate how far back in the encounter the hypothesis (or hypotheses) did occur, even returning the videotape to the beginning if necessary.

One very crucial point occurs just before the student gets up to examine the patient. At that point he should be asked the following questions.

1. "What was the patient's problem as you saw it then?"
2. "What specifically were you planning to do at this point?" The intent of this question is for him to describe exactly what items on physical examination were important to him as actions to sort out the ideas he had in his head about the patient's problem.
3. "What did you expect to find?" As an extension of the second question, this attempts to find out what ideas he had as to whether there would be positive or negative findings for specific items he wanted to examine.

It is important for the interviewer to ask questions whenever a change in the student's approach or thinking can be sensed on the videotape. As the videotape recall progresses, the interviewer should take notes concerning specific items that are to be evaluated. It would be valuable to make an audiotape of the recall interview, in case some sections have to be referred to again to clear up doubt or confusion as to what the student said.

This can be a very lengthy and time-consuming analysis. At the present time the authors are investigating the value of looking only at the first third of the encounter for an analysis of clinical reasoning, since the studies of physicians have shown that most hypotheses, inquiry strategies, and problem formulations have been completed by that time.

Self-Study Evaluation

Self-Evaluation

The first component of the student's self-study abilities to be evaluated is his ability for self-evaluation. How well does he review his work with the problem he has just encountered, to see if there are inadequacies in his knowledge or skills that require further work or study? To see if he has analyzed his ability in self-evaluation, the teacher can ask him specific questions in the following areas, either through direct examination, a write-up, or answers to structured questions on a form. The items do not necessarily have to follow this sequence.

Inquiry Path. Were the appropriate actions taken in the appropriate sequence? The student should be able to analyze this once he has completed his work with a problem and understood the mechanisms responsible for the problem or diagnosis. This can also be analyzed by the ratings given to his actions in particular problem formats, such as the P4, PMP, and some computer programs.

Hypotheses. Were these adequate, too specific, too vague, sufficiently inclusive to capture the important data, or appropriate for the educational goals with the problem? This latter refers to the error of making diagnostic hypotheses in a problem that was used to learn about underlying dysfunction or basic mechanisms.

Data Interpretation. Were the information and observations from the patient, tests, consultations, or other material perceived and correctly interpreted?

Problem Formulation. Was the problem formulation appropriate, did it contain too many extraneous details or facts, did it leave out significant positive or negative information, was it phrased in too biased a fashion that would push toward an unwarranted diagnostic hypothesis; were *all* problems identified in the formulation?

Diagnostic Decision. Was the correct hypothesis selected from those thought of, could other hypotheses have been selected, were they ranked correctly, was the diagnostic decision sensitive to likelihood or treatability of the possible disease processes?

Therapeutic Decisions (if appropriate). Were the correct choices made, were these decisions sensitive to the patient's needs or his psychosocial problems?

Sequential or Continuing Management. Were all new data appropriately utilized to change evaluative or treatment decisions?

Efficiency (if appropriate). Was the use of time, or the cost of the tests or procedures requested, appropriate?

If the student used an actual patient or simulated patient in his problem work, the following areas should be evaluated.

1. Appropriate use of clinical skills, interview, and examination
2. Appropriate use of interpersonal skills.

The student's use of available evaluative tools to help him in this assessment can be evaluated, such as a self-assessment unit, formulas as available in the PMP or P4, review and comparison of criterion performances as available, peer review, or review with faculty.

Design of Study Questions

Did the student use an educational prescription? Were educational issues identified that were unique to the particular problem with which he was working? Were the areas defined where additional learning was needed to complete or understand the problem? Was the student's focus for study appropriate to the problem? Were the priorities he set for self-study appropriate?

Use of Educational Resources

Were the correct resources used for the information he wished to acquire? Were they used correctly? Did he know how to use the library or resource lists appropriately? Did he know the appropriate use of the audiovisual media involved? Did he know how to contact and work with appropriate people in the faculty to gain his information?

Efficiency

The student's efficiency can be looked at, in terms of time spent and study accomplished.

New Knowledge Acquired

Another area of concern in self-study evaluation is the information gained by the student as a consequence of his self-study. To look purely at information gained may be somewhat crude when you look at the overall intent of problem-based learning but it is tested easily by the use of a variety of multiple-choice, true–false questions. Pre- and posttests are necessary if one is to accurately estimate information gained. Even more important, however, would be a look at the information or skills that have been acquired and applied back to the problem. This can be seen if the student revises his hypothesis, diagnostic or treatment decisions as a consequence of his study. His evaluation or critique of his clinical reasoning done before his self-directed study now might be sharper and more focused.

The most crucial step in self-directed study, mentioned in previous chapters, is the student's ability to generalize and synthesize the information and skills learned in his work with a problem. These points should be considered.

1. Has he used the information gained in his study to expand or improve upon his present understanding about the particular subject areas involved in his study?
2. Has his understanding of the anatomical (or other) area involved improved over his previous understanding?
3. How has he incorporated or synthesized this information into a whole?
4. Has he put the information gained regarding the problem into an overall model or system that might be useful for further reference?
5. Has he taken the information gained from the problem and generalized its possible applicability to future problems in similar areas in which the information might be helpful?

The evaluation of the student's self-directed study can be accomplished best on the basis of informal discussions, either with the student as an individual, or with a group if the students are involved in small-group learning. The questions just listed can be asked in such discussions. In addition, the teacher and the students can look at the individual's contribution to the group's understanding of the problem in the group process.

A more formal evaluation of self-directed study can be accomplished in the following way.

1. The student works through the self-directed study problem, without any break, until he has either concluded his work or feels he can go no further.
2. The student writes up the patient problem, including
   a. A data base containing all the information he feels is important in understanding the problem
   b. His formulation of the problem
   c. His hypotheses concerning the nature of the problem, in terms of either diagnosis or basic mechanisms
   d. Whatever treatment or management plans he feels would be appropriate.
3. The student is given a multiple-choice or true–false pretest for information base, if this is felt necessary.
4. The student then is allowed to carry out self-directed study in any manner he wishes for a prescribed period of time. (A variation of this is to provide the student with a room full of resources in which the self-directed study is to be carried out, if you wish to observe his study habits and the particular materials he uses.)
5. At the end of the self-directed study time, the student is given the opportunity to review his write-up and revise, as appropriate. This

gives an indication of how the new information he has gained has been applied to his work with the problem.

6. The multiple-choice or true–false posttest is given if necessary. This should include questions both related and unrelated to the problem, to avoid artificial cueing provided by the pretest obscuring a need to know defined by the encounter with the problem.

7. The student then writes a self-evaluation, in either a free or structured form, utilizing the points mentioned previously. The student is asked to list the resources used and to comment on the educational gains he has made.

8. The student is asked to write down his recommendations for future study, based on this experience.

Another formal method of evaluating the results of self-directed study is to give the student a second problem to work with after he has returned from his period of self-directed study, to see if the information or skills gained have improved his clinical reasoning. This works best in problem formats in which there is a variety of measurement tools that can be used, such as simulated patients, PMPs, or P4s, and where performance criteria can be specified carefully.

Setting Criteria and Scoring

There is extensive literature on the criteria for, and the scoring and analyzing of responses to multiple-choice and true–false questions. These should be referred to for the assessment of information recall.

In problem-based learning, the issue of evaluation concerns the *appropriate application of recalled information.* More important than measuring the student's ability to recall information, therefore, is the need to measure his cognitive skills; clinical reasoning; and the psychomotor skills of interview, examination, interpersonal communication, and treatment.

Clinical Reasoning Skills

Hard, measureable criteria are impossible in this area; however, criteria for performance can refer to the presence and quality of the various components of the clinical reasoning process, which are as follows.

1. Search for cues on relevant information
2. Multiple hypotheses generation; quality and adequacy
3. Inquiry strategies

4. Problem formulation
5. Hypothesis elimination or verification by deduction
6. Diagnostic decisions (or problem list)
7. Treatment decisions.

Evaluation of Clinical Reasoning with Specific Problems

Harder measurement can be developed if these components are looked at relevant to a specific problem with which the student is being evaluated and by specifying some or all of the following.

1. The cues that are important for the student to perceive at the beginning of the patient problem
2. The relevant data available in the patient problem (remember that physicians usually employ only 60 percent of this information in their reasoning)
3. The appropriate initial hypotheses, appropriate to the level of the student and appropriate to the setting in which the problem is being presented (See conceptual framework in Bashook, 1976)
4. The appropriate or adequate problem formulation
5. The important or crucial sequences in the inquiry strategy (clearly, some actions should occur before others; for example, a fundoscopic examination should be done before a lumbar puncture)
6. The appropriate diagnostic formulations (or appropriate problem list if the problem-oriented record is used)
7. The appropriate laboratory tests and their sequence
8. The appropriate treatment
9. The value of any action taken by the student toward work with the problem. The actions the students take can be scored by any of a variety of scales, depending on the type of problem situation. With the use of simulated patients, for example, the actions may have to be scored in retrospect.
10. The actions that would be relevant to all possible hypotheses associated with a problem. This is not exactly the same as the item number 9. Here, criteria are made as to the appropriate actions for any hypotheses entertained by the student encountering the problem. As a consequence, his sequence of actions then can be evaluated against the hypotheses he developed, correct or incorrect.

There are several problems in all of this. Who sets these criteria? If the problem is one that has been designed for clinical reasoning and learning in basic science, should the basic science faculty set these criteria or should they be set by physicians who are specialists in the area of the problem? Should basic scientists who have an M.D. degree set the criteria? Who is appropriate? If the problem is for students at the clinical level, should the criteria be set by specialists in the area of the problem, by general internists or surgeons (if it happens to be in appropriate areas), or by family physicians? Perhaps students, a year ahead of the student being evaluated with a particular problem format, should be involved in the setting of criteria. Perhaps house staff, such as interns and residents, should be involved. These are very difficult decisions that have to be made by the faculty on the basis of educational objectives and their particular educational philosophy about the appropriate evaluation and care of patients.

The next issue is how these criteria are to be set. Should one person be designated as a problem designer for a particular course, or should a curriculum committee be responsible for setting the criteria in consultation with the appropriate people on the faculty; Should a panel of experts be pulled together to set the criteria or should this be the result of an education committee or some other group?

The third and crucial problem in criteria setting is the fact that there really is no *one* right way to reason through or manage a problem. Although there can be clear constraints in the range of actions that are effective or efficient in the problem and in the range of hypotheses and formulations that are possible, there still is no one right way. The criteria have attempted to avoid prescribing a one right way. To help whoever is responsible by whatever mechanism to develop the criteria that are necessary, the documentation of "reference performances" often is helpful. A reference performance is the encounter between an identified expert on the faculty and the problem format used by the student. For example, a problem-based learning unit in neurology might be encountered by neurologists, family physicians, and clinical nurses, as appropriate. (The best approach, of course, would be to have all three reference performances available, to be used by the appropriate students in appropriate settings.) As a result of this encounter, the expert is asked to write up the problem in the form acceptable within a particular medical school. If it is a P4 or PMP, the flow of choices is recorded. It also would be valuable if a simulated patient were used, so a videotape could be made of the performance. Even if a simulated patient is not used, it is important to have the expert note down the initial problem formulation, the hypotheses generated, and some comments about their inquiry strategy. On the basis of this information, a far more realistic set of criteria for the student performance can be drawn up. Experience has not shown that criteria are more valuable when obtained in this manner, as opposed to having experts on the faculty review the problem as an intellectual exercise and describe what they feel the criteria should be. These reference performances also are useful in self-assessment units. They allow the student to compare his performance with the reference performance and evaluate his performance with regard to his particular level of learning.

In our experience with the development of problem-based units, we have found it to be most efficacious if one person is given the job of designing the criteria for performance. Although a panel of experts from the various areas is necessary, one person has to be the final authority. The mechanism for making these decisions should be specified ahead of time. In pulling together a series of problems in the neuroscience area, for example, the panel consisted of three neurologists, two neurological nurses, and three neuroscientists. In another setting in which criteria for simulated-patient assessments were being developed, the panel consisted of two specialists, two family physicians, and two faculty involved in the course in which the problems were used.

Such criteria are important for formative self-evaluation but are essential for summative evaluation using problems.

Clinical Skills

These can be evaluated in general or for a certain problem. Clinical skills evaluation forms are multitudinous. They usually request the observer to score the student on a scale of, for example, five choices for each separate observation about the student's clinical skills. Clarity in defining these criteria is particularly important. More focused observations, asking for scoring of specialized areas (for example, an aphasia interview, a pelvic examination, or a particular procedure) may be specified for particular problems.

Interpersonal Skills

There is a number of established tools that can be used by an observer in scoring the student's skills in this area. The faculty can specify what characteristics they wish the student to employ. If a simulated patient is used, forms can be designed for them to score their reaction to the student's skills. It is important to remember that the report of an appropriately trained simulated patient can be one of the most potent and accurate parts of the interpersonal skill assessment.

Bashook (1976) has offered a conceptual framework for the measuring of clinical problem solving, which can be adapted to the clinical reasoning process defined here. This framework is particularly valuable for problem-based learning because it defines three dimensions that need to be considered in setting criteria for competent performance.

1. The individual components of the problem-solving process
2. The specific clinical discipline or area with which the problem is encountered, such as medicine, surgery, psychiatry, gynecology, pediatrics, family medicine, and so forth
3. The specific context in which the care is being provided, such as acute or intensive care, chronic care, routine health maintenance, emergency room care, and the like.

The use of such a construct for each problem can be valuable, not only in setting the criteria for particular students in particular settings, but for determining who might provide the best "reference performance." Certainly the clinical reasoning process required for an emergency room patient for whom only a few quick, high-priority assessments can be allowed and for whom intervention is an immediate requirement, would be quite different from a patient with a chronic, intermittent problem. The approach to right upper quadrant pain in a surgical setting may be quite different from that for the same syndrome in a medical setting. These dimensions provide a tool both for analyzing the performance of experts working with your problem and for drawing up the criteria of competence for the student.

Process versus Outcome

It may be that we have become so preoccupied with hypothetical ideas about what constitutes good clinical skills and good interpersonal skills, through the use of evaluation forms, that we have lost sight of what really is important in medicine: the ability to evaluate and manage the patient's medical and psychosocial problem(s). In fact, the experience of evaluating a large number of excellent physicians working with simulated-patient problems has underlined this concern. Many of these physicians employed clinical skills and interpersonal techniques which would have given them a rather low score on the sanctimonious evaluation forms produced within the medical school; nevertheless, their diagnostic decisions and their treatment programs were most appropriate. In addition, the patient and/or simulated patient involved with that physician subsequently described their complete satisfaction with his ministrations and their willingness to return and comply.

We would suggest, therefore, that only four outcomes really matter in the interaction between a physician (or a student) and the patient, and that what actually goes on in the process is of no consequence in the evaluation of the student or physician if these four outcomes are satisfactory. They can be listed as follows.

1. An accurate assessment of the patient's problem should result, as accurate as available data allow, and no more accurate than data allow.
2. The management plan should be appropriate in terms of payoff, risk, and cost.
3. Time should be used efficiently. The clinician should not take an hour to evaluate a patient when it should take only 15 minutes.
4. The patient should be satisfied with the experience and be willing to comply or return to the student and/or physician, as appropriate. (If the patient is emotionally disturbed or unresponsive, this satisfaction would have to lie with a relative or responsible person associated with the patient.)

If these outcomes are met, it should not be important if the student stares at the ceiling, belches, asks weird questions, or holds a reflex hammer incorrectly. This returns us to our original objectives for medical school, where our greatest concern is that we produce physicians who are capable of evaluating and managing patients and their problems effectively, efficiently, and humanely. Process concerns may need to be developed in school, but certainly are not crucial in terms of assessing the student's abilities.

As mentioned previously, these outcomes are not true outcomes in terms of measuring whether the patient ultimately benefits or worsens; rather, they give us every reason to expect that the patient would profit from the student's or physician's performance (see discussion of process versus outcome earlier in this chapter).

How Many Problems Are Needed to Certify Competency?

The final problem in the evaluation of the clinical reasoning process and in the evaluation of medical students' competency to care for patients is that of predictive validity. If our principal objective is for students to be able to evaluate and manage patients' medical problems effectively, efficiently, and humanely, then how do we certify that this objective has been met by the student? How can we certify that he is capable of independent patient practice or able to continue to educate himself?

We have considered the tools that would allow us to assess the whole range of student capability with any particular problem; however, the student's ability to evaluate and manage one problem successfully is an unreliable measure of his skill. He might have had a recent or extensive experience with that kind of problem, or he might have made some lucky guesses. If he did well with that problem, would he do well with one in another area of medicine? If the problem he worked with was an inpatient problem, how would he do with an outpatient problem? If the problem was simple, how would he do with a complicated problem, an emergency problem, a chronic problem, or a problem with psychogenic overlay? This underlines the three dimensions described by Bashook (1976).

The first decision for the faculty is to determine exactly with which problems the student should be competent, and how competent he should be. This would be different for a graduate from medical school than it would be for a graduate from a residency training program. The setting of criteria for competency has been discussed already. The next decision is to determine *how many* problems and *what variety* should be used to predict the student's performance. Research has failed, thus far, to answer this question. It is obvious only that more than one should be used, and that the more that can be employed in the student's evaluation the more reliable the predictions will become.

In conclusion, there is a whole range of powerful evaluation tools that can be used by students and teachers in problem-based learning to look at the intermediate steps and the total product of the clinical reasoning process, including the following.

1. Time-out discussions during the use of simulated patients, P4s, PMPs, and the like; dissecting the student's thought processes
2. Videotape review sessions of thinking with real or simulated patients, looking at segments of the clinical reasoning process and the information brought to the problem
3. Observing a student with real and simulated patients
4. Feedback from simulated patients about the student's interpersonal skills.

These can be used as frequently as needed as a personal tool for both student and faculty to diagnose and treat educational needs of students. When more reliable measurements are needed, criteria can be developed by group concensus. These need to be reviewed and altered, as appropriate, as more student experience is gained with them. Criteria can be developed by the student himself from "reference performances."

CHAPTER 8

Selection of the Appropriate Problems for Learning

The advantages of problem-based learning in medical education, the methods for carrying it out in a variety of educational settings and levels, and ways to evaluate problem-based learning have been discussed. This included a consideration of the formats or methods for presenting the patient problem to students, ranging from card decks through specially trained people. The choice of format depends on the specific educational objectives at the time. The next issue that must be considered is the variety or types of patient problems that should be simulated for an educational program and how many should be simulated.

The faculty or teacher of problem-based learning does not necessarily have to give to the students problems that represent classical diseases or disorders. They rarely occur in reality. The patient problems presented can be complex, vague, undiagnosed, or simple, as long as they achieve the learning felt appropriate. In the students' attempt to discover what mechanisms are responsible or what diseases are possible, they will learn about diseases in the appropriate context. It is important to present the students with problems as they appear in reality.

It also would defeat the advantages of problem-based learning if problems representing known disease entities were labeled or identified as such. Patients never come to the physician with the disease written on their foreheads. The physician's task is to disentangle and identify the patient's problem. Although our discussion here will refer to diseases, disorders, or symptom complexes, all problems will be presented to the student as an unknown to be resolved.

The easiest method for determining what problems need to be identified and produced is to have the faculty in a particular discipline or section of the curriculum put together into one document all the information and skills that they feel should be learned. This is the method used to create the "problem boxes" for a neuroscience course (Barrows & Mitchell, 1975). A survey was made of all the concepts taught in a variety of integrated neuroscience courses around the United States and Canada. This was assembled on a master chart. It listed all the important content areas taught in neuroanatomy, neurophysiology, neurochemistry, neuropharmacology, neuropathology, clinical neurology, and physical neurological diagnoses. Well-documented neurological patient problems then were selected at random from clinical records. The information that self-directed study areas should cover with each problem was checked off the list. For example, a case of multiple sclerosis featuring many neurological deficits, including a blind eye and paraplegia, led to the coverage of the following items.

1. Spinal cord localization
2. Spinal cord anatomy; ascending and descending pathways
3. Bladder control and function
4. "Spinal shock"
5. Babinski reflex
6. Motor examination
7. Sensory examination
8. Examination of vision
9. Physiology of vision
10. Myelin; anatomy and function
11. Demyelinating diseases
12. Transverse myelitis.

As subsequent patient problems were selected, many of the same items would be checked off again, as well as new items. In a case of myasthenia gravis, the following additional items were checked off.

1. Physiology, pharmacology, and anatomy of the myoneural junction
2. Evaluation of extraocular muscle function
3. Motor examination
4. Immunological diseases involving the nervous system.

This continued until, by the 22nd problem, the last items were checked off. It was assumed, therefore, that the assembled problems should have been able to lead the students into almost any area of neuroscience learning on the basis of self-directed study.

The student groups were able, with the help of their faculty "tutor" and occasional advice from the course planners, to choose from the list the problems most relevant for their learning. Several years' experience showed that student groups tended to pick those problems most frequently present in general practice situations. It also was found that they were involved in areas of learning far beyond those anticipated for each problem. As a consequence, they achieved a firm foundation in the neuroscience knowledge needed to handle the common problems. In no instance did any group have either the time or inclination to take on all 22 problems; however, some carried out brief encounters with the remaining problems at the end of the course, to see what unique features they offered that might need to be reviewed.

To help them in their self-directed study, the students were provided with a document that listed the neurological problems and concepts that a group of neurological educators from around North America felt should be understood by a medical student on graduation, regardless of his ultimate specialty or career. In addition, the students saw many demonstrations with real patients and had opportunities for personal work with patients, so they could transfer into practice what they had to learn.

A second method, utilized by a group designing a problem-based approach for the education of physicians and nurses in the evaluation and care of neonatal respiratory failure, represents a more focused approach (Barrows et al., 1978). Although it was aimed at postgraduate and continuing medical education, it seems very relevant for any specialty area, particularly one such as neonatal respirology, which is a new, rapidly advancing field in which limited learning resources are available. This group chose neonatal respiratory problems that fulfilled the following criteria:

1. Those problems most commonly seen
2. Those problems poorly handled in the community, as determined by survey of neonates referred to a center for specialized care
3. Those problems that would emphasize important or new concepts in neonatal care
4. Those problems that require early identification because they are treatable and because intervention can significantly reduce mortality or morbidity.

Some of the problems were developed so that they could be followed in order. A sequence of problem units (P4s) was designed for one problem: (1) the mother early in her pregnancy, (2) the mother at delivery, and (3) the neonate at delivery.

This gave them the problems that seemed necessary to learning the contemporary evaluation and care of neonates with respiratory difficulties.

Their next step was to consider each of these problems in turn and list the information and skills that would be needed to evaluate and care for each problem. They then condensed this into a second list of all the information and skills that any physician and nurse (or student, for that matter) might need in order to be competent with these neonates. The first list showed exactly which kind of patient problems needed to be simulated. The second list determined the kinds of learning resources that needed to be found, compiled, or produced.

The third method of selecting problems is probably the most appropriate and widely applicable to any curriculum or course that needs to select problems for problem-based learning. Teachers or faculty need to determine which problems in their area meet the following characteristics:

1. Problems, conditions, or diseases that have the greatest frequency in the usual practice setting
2. Those problems that represent life-threatening or urgent situations that require skillful, effective, emergency management
3. Those problems with a potentially serious outcome, in terms of morbidity or mortality, in which intervention – preventive or therapeutic – can make a significant difference in prognosis
4. Those problems most often poorly handled by physicians in the community, usually determined by surveying both specialists in hospitals or in other referral settings, as well as primary-care physicians. The latter group can be asked about the problems they feel give them the most difficulty in care
5. Those problems that emphasize or underline important concepts in basic sciences, such as anatomy, physiology, biochemistry, pathology, pharmacology, epidemiology, and so forth, necessary to give the student a sound foundation or prepare him for new trends or concepts in medicine.

These criteria for problem selection are aimed at the first-stated educational objective: effective and efficient patient care by the physician. The College of Family Practice of Canada uses a similar approach to determine what emphasis should be given to learning about any particular disorder in medical education. It gives each condition a score from one to five for each of three different characteristics: frequency, potential seriousness, and the effectiveness of intervention. These scores are multiplied together and the product determines the position of each condition on a list, showing the emphasis it should receive. Meningitis, for example, receives a low-frequency score of one, a potential-seriousness score of five, and a treatability score of five (Murray, 1977).

It could be reasoned that if the first four criteria are well met, the fifth really is not needed; however, this input from basic science faculty can suggest selection criteria for each problem that would emphasize their educational concerns better. For example, if it were felt that an acute encephalopathy in the child was an important problem from the standpoint of the clinicians, the biochemist might suggest that an illness, a Reye's syndrome with the problems of hypoglycemia and hepatic enzyme dysfunction, would be a useful challenge for student learning in a biochemical area he feels is important. This team approach in problem selection allows for the production of problems that have visibility with basic scientists and encourage them to lead students into appropriate self-directed learning in the basic sciences. The basic-sciences faculty can provide the student with learning resources appropriate to their self-directed learning (or teacher-directed learning) during work with the problem.

Since many disorders, diseases, or presenting problems may cover several criteria at once, the list of needed problems may not be as long as might be suggested by these many criteria. The odessy of Murray (1977) in attempting to define those problems needed to teach neurology is an excellent example of how one specialty thought through this problem. It is well worth reviewing.

Although this book deals principally with the design of *patient* problems, the professional task of most physicians, it is important to have problem-based learning resources in other areas. A P4 format was designed by Sinclair (1978) to help students at postgraduate or masters levels to evaluate their ability to design clinical trials. A sociopolitical problem, concerning environmental methyl-mercury in an autochthonous native population, was designed by the authors as part of an ongoing assessment of medical school applicants. A P4 format has been designed to teach biology students how to carry out genetic experimentation with fruit flies. Such research problems in P4, PMP, or computer formats would be very effective in helping students develop appropriate scientific reasoning skills and to evaluate the contribution of research to their clinical work. Many problems could be designed involving populations, laboratory tests, disease control, evaluation of experimental results, experimental design, and the like. Journal articles and drug company brochures also could be used as problem-based learning tools to challenge the student's ability to analyze research papers and reviews.

With all of this concern that appropriate problems are selected to cover the important problems in health care and the important information and skills in the clinical and basic science areas, it is important not to lose sight of the objective of problem-based, and particularly student-centered, learning.

For example, despite the existence of the 22 problem boxes in neurology that were assembled to cover all the important concepts of neurology and neuroscience in undergraduate medicine, the designers of the course were happy if the students worked through 6 (Barrows & Mitchell, 1975). The educational goals for this course were specified as follows.

> When confronted by a patient, or various representations of patients (protocol, slides, films, video tapes, simulated patients), the student should be able to:
> a) Obtain appropriate medical information or data concerning the problem by observation and examination as appropriate (examination of patient, simulated patients, observation of slides, films, audio tapes, etc.)
> b) Define the patient's problem or problems
> c) Describe the appropriate anatomical, physiological, psychological, pathological, biological information
> d) Describe how the suspected underlying pathophysiology might be verified by further investigations.

Despite the fact that all 22 problems would provide the student with a comprehensive base, the goals clearly were related to the development of clinical reasoning skills. The intent was for the student to gain an understanding of how the nervous system is put together and works and how to approach problems in the nervous system effectively, not to gain an encyclopedic knowledge. The student groups used educational prescriptions to guide in their choice of problems and the areas of self-study. The first few problems always required rather extensive study of terminology, anatomy, physiology, and the clinical concepts of examination and localization. It was felt that if the students studied only six problems well they would have gained an understanding and experience sufficient to allow them to tackle any further neurological problem and to build on the knowledge acquired by appropriate self-study. The effectiveness of a few problems in allowing the students to learn a great range of information has been a repeated experience of many teachers.

These methods of determining the problems that need to be designed or assembled for a program or course will allow a sufficient range of problems to be available to meet the individual learning needs of any student or student group at any level, depending upon their personal career goals, ability, and background knowledge. Enough problems are developed to allow some to be used for other purposes, such as review, elective experiences, and updating in postgraduate and continuing medical education. The teacher may set aside some time to be used in evaluation.

As a final thought, very effective student learning is derived from asking students to produce problem-based learning units for other students. This also is a mechanism for producing new units. It takes considerable study and scholarship to put together a problem in a simulation format and to provide evaluation tools. In addition, it introduces the student to educational concerns: objectives, technique, and evaluation.

CHAPTER 9

The Design of Problem-Based Learning Units

Having come this far in the book, the reader must have some well-developed convictions about the design of problem-based learning units. These units should provide a patient simulation in a format constructed to allow the student to interact with the patient problem in a manner that will both challenge and develop his clinical reasoning skills and stimulate his self-directed (or teacher-directed study). Problem-based learning units should also facilitate the student's ability to evaluate his skills and knowledge in working with the problem.

Elstein et al. (1972) have pointed out that an important characteristic of the challenge that patient problems offer the physician is that all the information needed to solve the problem is typically unavailable at the outset. All problem-based learning units should provide this challenge. This and other characteristics for educationally useful simulations have been identified by McGuire & Babbott (1967). The following list is an adaptation and expansion of their requirements for simulations.

1. The problem should be presented with the type of information normally available to the physician at the outset, not a predigested summary containing information that usually would result only from further inquiry by the physician.
2. The problem format should allow for sequential, interdependent actions to be taken in the evaluation and treatment of the patient problem.
3. The student should be provided with immediate information, in a realistic form, regarding the results of these actions.

4. The student should not be able to retract an action that is revealed to be ineffective or harmful.
5. The format should allow for different approaches to the patient's problem that lead to different outcomes as a result of different skills, strategies, or styles.
6. The design of the problem also should allow the student to practice and evaluate the important stages or segments of the clinical reasoning process, including
   a. Data perception and interpretation
   b. Problem formulation
   c. Hypothesis generation
   d. Inquiry strategy
   e. Diagnostic and therapeutic decisions
   f. Sequential management.
7. The units should incorporate as much visual and auditory representations as can be *conveniently* featured by the use of photographs, slides, films, audio and video tapes of patients, X rays, specimens, and the like.
8. Feasibility or ease of use by the student, as well as cost and reproduceability, must be considered.

Portable Patient Problem Pack (P4)

The P4, a fairly recent addition to the simulation armamentarium, is an example of how all these concerns and criteria might be considered in a problem-based learning resource (Barrows & Tamblyn, 1977).

Description

The P4 is a method of simulating a patient's problem in a card-deck format. It allows the student to take any action possible with the real patient and in the sequence he feels appropriate. As in the real clinical situation, the student is able to see the result of each action before deciding on the next. He is as free to make mistakes, perform unnecessary tests, or order incorrect treatments as he is to manage effectively the problem presented. As a result, the student can apply his problem-solving or diagnostic skills in a manner consistent with the clinical reasoning skills of the practicing clinician (characterized in Chapter 2).

Because it is a deck of cards, the P4 is a portable, easily used format that requires only a table top for use and does not require complex audiovisual hardware. It can be adapted to present the limitations and challenges of a variety of health-care settings: urban, rural, and remote. Any of the tests, procedures, consultants, or treatments that would not be available locally can be removed from the deck, allowing the student to work in the real task environment. In his work with the P4, the student also is able to observe and interpret X rays, electrocardiograms, fundoscopic appearances, histological specimens, and other items he might request in his work with real patient problems. Some problems do make use of audiovisual equipment, so that the student may see the patient's appearance in photographs, hear the patient being interviewed on audiotapes, and see the patient being evaluated on videotape.

A complete P4 unit, simulating one patient problem, consists of a deck of several hundred 3" X 5" cards in a variety of colors, a collection of 3" X 5" photographs, printed instructions, and evaluation materials. Colors categorize the type of action that can be taken with the patient, as shown in Table 9-1. On the front of each card, the specific action that the card represents is described in capital letters, some examples of which are shown in Table 9-2. Below this title is a series of questions that the student should ask himself, until it becomes automatic, before selecting any more cards of that color. Some examples are shown in Table 9-3. Note how these questions are designed to help shape the effectiveness and efficiency of the student's problem-solving or clinical reasoning skills. Cards for such actions as investigations and consultations have a time delay indicated that prevents the student from obtaining the results sooner than they would be available in real life.

The backs of the cards give the student the responses to the action indicated on the front: answers to questions, findings on physical examination, results of investigations, opinions of consultants, and results of intervention that actually occurred with the patient on whom the simulation was based or would have occurred if such action had been taken. Some of the backs refer the student to appropriate photographs of X rays, fundoscopic views, or laboratory or diagnostic tests, for him to observe and interpret. The

Table 9-1. Categories of action as denoted by card color in the P4 unit.

Color of card	Action category
White	Interview questions
Blue	Items on physical examination
Orange	Investigations, laboratory tests, and diagnostic procedures
Green	Consultants
Pink	Interventions, both medical and nursing
Yellow	"Situation" and "closure"

Table 9-2. Three examples of card titles, in each of three color categories, for individual actions selected from a P4 series in neurology.

History cards (white)

HOW DID YOUR PROBLEM START AND WHEN?
ANY PRECIPITATING OR AGGRAVATING FACTORS
  TO YOUR PROBLEM?
DOUBLE VISION?

Physical examination cards (blue)

VITAL SIGNS
CAROTID PULSES & SOUNDS
STRETCH REFLEXES

Investigative cards (orange)

BLOOD SUGAR
BLOOD ELECTROLYTES
CEREBRAL ANGIOGRAPHY

Table 9-3. Examples of the standardized questions that appear on the fronts of P4 cards, aimed at shaping students' problem-solving skills.

History cards (white)

Problem formulation?
Hypotheses?
Information needed?
  interview
  examinations
  investigations
  consultations
Study needed?
Next move?

Physical examination cards (blue)

Why select this card?
Could you perform this examination?
Can you interpret the possible results from this examination?
How would a positive or negative result influence your
  hypotheses?
Do you understand the principles or facts in human biology
  necessary to evaluate any findings?

interpretation of these materials is on the cards' backs, printed upside down to prevent accidental perception by the student before he has made his own observations.

The first card used, the "situation" card, initiates work with the problem. When turned over, it describes where the patient presents himself (emergency room, office, or clinic) and offers a brief statement of the presenting problem. The "closure" card is selected by the student to signify that he is finished and that he has made, in his mind, the appropriate diagnostic and treatment decisions. After he has drawn this card, no further cards can be drawn. The back side of this card asks a variety of questions the student should be able to answer if he has evaluated and understood the patient problem as presented. A separate series of "patient progress" cards allows the student to follow up on the patient's problem, over time, in the manner of a problem box or sequential management problem.

There are many more actions (cards) available in each deck than are necessary for, or even relevant to, the particular problem, thus permitting the student to take almost any conceivable action possible with the patient. This large number of cards and their specific titles *remain constant* in each P4 unit in any particular series of patient problems within one discipline. This minimizes the effect of cueing in a specific patient problem, since every card is always present, whether useful or not. The fronts of the cards and their number do not differentiate one patient problem from another. The backs for each deck are totally different, as they represent the responses and results of actions for one specific patient problem.

How the P4 Is Used

The student spreads the cards out in front of him so that all the titles can be seen, reads the back of the situation card, and acquaints himself with the problem. He decides which action he should take first, draws the appropriate card, reads the result, and then continues in this manner until he has decided that the problem has been handled as far as he can, or wishes, to carry it. If the unit is being used for problem-based learning, the student may stop at any time to read, study, or confer with faculty, before continuing with the deck. As he continues to work with the deck, he makes a pile with each card drawn placed on top of the previous cards he has chosen. At the end, the pile of cards represents his cognitive path and, as mentioned before, can be used to evaluate his skills in a variety of ways.

Range of Uses

The P4 can be utilized by individual students, pairs of students, groups of students, and classes, in a variety of interdisciplinary student teams. The deck and its play can be altered, depending upon the specific educational objectives of either the faculty or students involved.

The design of this simulation format allows it to be used for a variety of educational purposes, including (1) developing the student's cognitive skills in problem solving or clinical reasoning, (2) facilitating problem-based learning as an active educational process in acquiring both basic science and clinical knowledge and concepts related to the problem presented, (3) encouraging the development of self-directed study skills, and (4) providing tools for either the student or the faculty to use in evaluating the student's skills in effectively managing a specific patient problem.

Since the P4 simulates the patient in a very flexible format, it can be adapted easily to meet a variety of student needs at all levels of education in medicine, nursing, and other health professions, as well as in interdisciplinary team learning. Although designed to be used as a unit in a curriculum that features problem-based learning in small groups, it can be used in any educational program.

Scoring

Each P4 contains a "score" card for each color or action category. This card assigns a value, on a 2+ to 2− weighted scale, for each card in its color category, as determined by a panel of physicians and nurses who are actively practicing in the discipline from which the problems were selected. This score rates the appropriateness or relevance of the action described on the card in working with the patient's problem. Together with the data from an "inventory" card that described the total number of cards available with 2+, 1+, 0, 1−, and 2− values contained in each deck, formulas can be used to calculate the student's economy of actions, his proficiency, and how problem-oriented his actions were when compared with the score he would have obtained if his card selection were random. Some examples of these formulas are given in Table 9-4. These are aimed at providing objective measures of the student's problem-solving skills. Additional insight or information can be gained about the student's reasoning process by reviewing the number, sequence, and specific actions chosen in his work with the problem. These sequences can be compared with those chosen by peers and experts who have worked with the same P4.

The cards for investigations and consultants have the cost indicated on their backs. The cost of the individual student's approach with the patient can be calculated.

Printed materials that accompany the P4 include instructions, case write-ups, and card sequences chosen by a variety of health professionals. A list of issues have been included that, in the opinion of the variety of faculty in the basic and clinical sciences who have reviewed the deck, could be

Table 9-4. Scoring formulas for Use in the P4

*These formulas were designed to give a numerical value for student perform-
ance with respect to quantity of cards selected (economy), quality of performance (proficiency), and relevance to the problem (on and off target).
They also supply a tool with which to compare future work and progress with
other P4 problems, and to compare student performance with experts and
peers. These values are specifically designed for comparative evaluation. They
have no significance by themselves.*

A. Overall economy formula

$$1 - \frac{\text{number of cards selected}}{\text{number of cards available}}$$

The overall *economy formula* gives a score involving the number of cards
chosen to work up this patient in relation to the total number of cards
available. This is a quantitative score and does not include "quality" in the
work-up, but is concerned with economy of actions. With a maximum
score of 1, the students can compare how economical they were in the
patient work-up.

B. Clinical skills economy formula

$$1 - \frac{\text{number of history and physical cards selected}}{\text{number of history and physical cards available}}$$

Clinical skills economy is also a quantitative measurement. It allows the
student to look at the extent to which he uses the history and physical
examination of a patient to arrive at an initial impression and management
plan. As with the overall economy score, a maximum of 1 can be obtained.

C. Proficiency formula

$$\frac{[2(+2 \text{ sel.}) + (+1 \text{ sel.})] - [2(-2 \text{ sel.}) + (-1 \text{ sel.})]}{\text{number selected}}$$

The proficiency formula is one assessment of the "quality" of the work-up
of a patient. It incorporates and weighs both the good and bad actions and
cards taken with this problem. A maximum score of 2 can be reached. The
+2 and −2 cards are given twice the weight as the +1 and −1 cards.

D. On-target formula

$$\frac{+2 \text{ cards selected}}{\text{number of cards selected}} - \begin{array}{l}\text{"random" score appropriate}\\\text{for the number of cards}\\\text{chosen (listed on the}\\\text{inventory card)}\end{array}$$

(continued)

Table 9–4. *(continued)*

D. On-target formula *(continued)*

The on-target formula represents a second assessment of the quality of the patient work-up. It determines the degree to which the selection of cards is directly relevant to the patient problem. This will give an idea of the appropriateness of choices to the problem. The scoring system (+2) on the score cards will assist in determining the score. Once this value is determined, subtract the random score for the total number of cards selected. This can be found on the inventory card. This will indicate how much more relevant or problem-oriented the student performance was than random selection of the cards.

E. Off-target formula

$$\frac{-2 \text{ cards selected}}{\text{number of cards selected}} - \begin{array}{l}\text{``random'' score appropriate}\\ \text{for the number of cards}\\ \text{selected (listed on the}\\ \text{inventory card)}\end{array}$$

The off-target formula is the last form of assessment of the quality of the work-up. It determines the degree to which the work-up is incompetent, costly, or dangerous to the patient. Again, subtract the appropriate random score for the total number of cards selected. Random scores for off-target for between 10 and 100 cards selected are provided on the inventory card.

studied profitably by the student during self-directed learning. A variety of approaches to evaluation are thus available to faculty or students.

Patient Progress Pack (P3)

The P3 is a sequential management problem in a separate deck of buff-colored cards enclosed with each P4. The P3 allows the student to follow the patient's progress over time. With each card the student can write down any reformulation of the patient's problem that he feels is appropriate and note any new actions, history taking, physical examinations, investigations, consultations, or management he would like to perform. In this way, the student can compare his approach with that of the clinicians who had managed the patient's problem.

The front card contains the instructions for work with the P3. Subsequent cards contain statements about crucial points in the patient's clinical course (new findings on history and examination and the results of investigations). With each card, the student can commit himself on paper as to how he would evaluate the new information he has obtained about the patient and how he would manage the patient before going on to the next card. As this is a sequential management format, each new card reveals how those who were responsible for the patient actually did evaluate and manage the patient at that point in time. Since the student makes his decisions before viewing the next card, he can evaluate these decisions in the continued care of the patient before he finds out what actions actually were undertaken.

Additional P4 Materials

The P4 itself is a pack of cards. Associated with the pack, to complete the problem unit, is a variety of other materials, some already mentioned, which include the following.

Photographs. These are the same size as the cards and are numbered on their backs for reference. They may be reproductions of the patient's appearance, physical signs, X rays, computerized tomography scans, brain scans, electroencephalograms, electrocardiograms, and the like, as appropriate for the particular patient. They may show *normal* or *abnormal* findings.

Audiotapes. These are compact cassettes and, when present in the P4 system, may feature an interview with the patient or present a sample of the patient's speech if it demonstrates pathology important for evaluation. In this latter instance, the tape will be referred to on the back of the appropriate card.

Videotapes. If present, they show the patient being worked up by a clinician, a physician, or a nurse; they are keyed to the appropriate cards.

Patient's Prior Health Records. These records, if present, can be used to provide past medical information on the patient. They also can be used as prior practice records, if the student wishes to take on the patient in a primary care or family medicine setting.

Consultation Reports. These reports expand on the opinions of some clinicians or consultants who have worked with the patient problem. They provide more information than is printed on the backs of appropriate green cards. These reports can be used best as a criterion by which the student's write-up of the patient can be assessed. In this way, the accuracy of the student's own problem formulation, data base, and management plan can be evaluated.

P4 Flows.   The sequence of cards chosen by the practicing clinicians, family physicians, nurses, and neurologists, who also took on the P4 as an unknown, is listed. This provides yet another opportunity for the student to compare his approach to the patient's problem with an expert's performance, cards chosen, and sequence chosen. Their evaluation formulas also can be calculated, for comparison.

Issues.   This booklet lists the possible educational issues that could arise from study about the particular patient problem featured. The list is compiled by faculty from many disciplines in both basic and clinical science. Each has listed the possible areas of learning in his own discipline that would be relevant to understanding or managing the patient's problem. This manual is designed to help the student with his self-directed study. The booklet probably is best referred to after the student has finished his own self-directed studies related to the patient problem. It serves as a guide for evaluation of the adequacy of the student's own study focus, and can suggest profitable areas of study that may not have occurred to the student.

Data Base.   This is a concise summary of all the data in the patient problem: data available on history, physical examination, and laboratory or diagnostic studies. It also summarizes the patient's progress in the P3. It is included primarily as a guide for faculty in helping them adapt the P4 to their particular educational program or course.

Evaluation of the Student's P4 Learning

An essential aspect of any problem-based learning unit is evaluation. The problem-based learning or problem-simulation format should allow the student, student groups, or faculty to evaluate the student's reasoning, knowledge base, applications of knowledge, and self-study skills. The features built into the P4 unit are described again here, to show how concerns for evaluation affect design.

Evaluation of Problem Solving or Clinical Reasoning

Standardized Questions.   The questions on the card fronts challenge the student's reasoning with each action taken. Answered mentally or verbally, they provide the student with an idea of the adequacy of both the knowledge he has to apply to this problem and his clinical reasoning skills. If he cannot answer these questions easily, a learning need is identified. Although potent, evaluation such as this is not measured easily.

Scoring. The student can record the cards he has selected, in the sequence they were selected, by using their identification number. Score cards of matching color list the value assigned for each of the cards he has selected. These values can be recorded opposite the identification number. Assigned by a panel of experienced clinicians, they range on a scale of +2 to −2, based on the following criteria.

+2   Indicates an appropriate choice of action with this patient's problem.

+1   Indicates that this choice is not related directly to defining or managing the patient's problem. If a comprehensive evaluation is appropriate, however, this card is valuable. The appropriateness of such an evaluation depends upon objectives or the amount of time available with the patient.

 0   Indicates a choice that has no effect one way or the other. Although it does not contribute to an understanding of the patient's problem, it is not expensive, inconvenient, or uncomfortable for the patient.

−1   Indicates a choice that is clearly unrelated to an effective approach to the patient's problem and may be expensive, uncomfortable, or dangerous to the patient.

−2   Indicates a choice that, in addition to being of no value to understanding or managing the patient's problem, is excessively expensive, time consuming, painful, or definitely dangerous to the welfare of the patient.

Formula Cards

Using the formulas listed on the formula card and the values assigned to the cards, the student can score various aspects of his clinical reasoning. These numbers can be used to assess progress in subsequent P4's. They provide a measureable score for problem solving.

Closure Cards

General questions are listed on the back of the closure card, which the student should be able to answer after he has completed the P4 and P3. If the student chooses a specific educational focus for work with the P4, he may find that only a few of the questions may be appropriate for his goals.

Cost Efficiency

The cost of the student work-up with the problem can be calculated by adding up the costs on the back of the orange and green cards selected. If the patient was admitted, the additional costs for the number of days he was kept in hospital, using hospitalization costs typical of the area, can be added.

P4 Flows

The student can compare his P4 flow (the sequence and number of cards selected) with those of expert clinicians who, like the student, took the problem on as an unknown. He can compare his selection of cards and his hypotheses with theirs. The student can see if this gives him insight about possibly better approaches than those he employed.

The students can compare their P4 flow with those of their peers. Much can be learned from the differences in their approaches and discussion of the reasoning behind these approaches.

Problem Write-Up

The student can compare his write-up of the problem with those written by reference clinicians. Are his data or his interpretations different? If so, why? He can compare both data base, evaluation, and management plan.

Self-Study

Another important design feature for problem-based learning units is the facilitation of self-directed study. The units help the student define areas of knowledge where further study may be indicated. The student is given the following suggestions with the P4 units.

1. Before starting the P4, decide what general area(s) you wish to con-centrate on in your self-study, such as physiology, diagnostic investi-gations, anatomy, patient management, epidemiology, and so forth.
2. As you work with the P4, note on a sheet of paper any information or skills you feel you lack or need to review, any holes in your knowledge, or any areas of confusion. This will act as a guide to your self-study.
3. As you play the P4, discipline yourself to answer mentally the ques-

tions on the card front. They will help you determine the adequacy of your knowledge and skills at any time during play and will suggest areas of profitable study.

4. If you get to a point in your P4 play where it is difficult to continue selecting appropriate cards on the basis of your present knowledge, you should stop and formulate a study plan.

5. Return to the P4 after study and apply to the problem the information you have learned. Continue until you feel you have completed your work, depending on your goals.

6. After completing the P4, *summarize* what new information you have learned (facts, principles), how this relates to what you already know, and how it will help you with similar problems in the future. After completing your self-study as related to the problem presented, be sure to review the issues that have been defined by expert consultants in the area you have studied, You will find these in booklets accompanying the P4 system. Their questions may indicate other subject areas you could pursue in your study of this problem, depending on your educational goals.

Note how these instructions to the student shape his study structure, just as the questions on the card fronts shape his reasoning.

Flexibility

This allows a learning resource to be adapted easily to meet the needs of a variety of students, educational objectives, and teaching–learning situations. Because they represent simulations of a patient problem, the formats should be useful in any situation in which a patient could be used in learning or evaluation, at any educational level from high school through continuing medical education.

With the P4, the student can meet clinical goals by using a simulated patient trained to simulate the problem in the deck. This challenges his skills in interview and examination and his interpersonal skills. After his contact with the simulated patient, he can eliminate the history and physical cards and work with the investigation, consultant, and management cards, as well as the P3, to continue with the problem. Videotapes of the actual patient or a simulated patient can challenge the student's clinical observation skills. An audiotape can present the patient being interviewed. If skills are required for more remote health-care settings, the student can remove from the P4 the consultants and more exotic tests that would not be available. To teach or evaluate efficiency in patient assessment and management, the student can be limited in the number of cards he can select. The student must select only the actions essential to understanding and dealing with the presenting problem, thus approximating the emergency situation where there is limited time for patient evaluation and management. To meet clinical or basic science goals, the student could use the P4 in a number of ways.

In summary, the following are offered as examples of the great number of possible educational uses.

1. To understand the underlying anatomy or pathophysiology of the problem presented, the student could concentrate on hypotheses and formulations of altered pathophysiology, in order to decide eventually on the underlying mechanisms involved in the patient problem.

2. To understand the basis and use of a variety of laboratory investigations, the student could enter the problem by reading the data base and summarizing the clinical findings. He then could use the investigation cards to analyze the problem and suggest self-study areas.

3. To improve skills in nursing management, the student might read the data base, which summarizes the significant findings on history, physical, and lab investigations, and then use the pink and green cards to select an appropriate management plan.

4. To meet interdisciplinary (medicine and nursing) goals, the P4 can be used as the stimulus for study and discussion among students or health professionals from different disciplines. Working as a group, they can use experience and knowledge from their own discipline to contribute to an understanding and resolution of the problem. In addition, they can identify individual study areas that are compatible with their career goals and would be useful in helping them deal with this and future problems. Each discipline group, in the process of dealing with a patient problem, has the opportunity to sort out its professional roles without the responsibility and pressure present in the actual patient situation.

As an example, a continuing medical education program has been mounted by the neonatal program at McMaster University, focusing on the treatment of neonatal respiratory distress (Barrows et al., 1978). The program is aimed at the nurses and physicians who care for high-risk mothers and premature infants in remote and rural hospital settings. Using a series of P4s that present problems common in this area, nurses and physicians in each hospital meet locally to work through these problems, identifying learning needs as necessary for a collaborative attempt at a resolution of the problem. Informal feedback to date indicates that this approach is an interesting and rewarding challenge for the participants.

Media

It is necessary to consider how the media should be employed in problem-based learning units to enhance the reality of the patient problem and to challenge visual or auditory observations by students. There are several aspects of media that need to be considered.

Appropriateness

The choice of audiotapes, photographs, slides, videotapes, film, or three-dimensional stereoscopic slides depends on the information to be transferred. Audiotapes should be used for patient interview, speech, or manner of verbal expression. Videotapes or films are required for observation of patient gaits, movement disorders, cine-radiographs, procedures, operations, or interview and examination of the patient. Slide transparencies or photographs are used for images that are static, such as X rays, scans, histological slides, hematological slides, patient appearance, fundi, skin lesions, clinic sites, environmental data, living conditions, and so on. Stereoscopic slides can be used for dysmorphic or skeletal changes, such as muscle atrophy. The media selected always must be appropriate to the information being conveyed. Abstract concepts, introductory and background information, static images, and lectures should not be presented on videotape. Small print and detailed diagrams should not go on slides. A patient should not be described in print.

Convenience to the Student

If the audiovisual material can be used easily, without gadgets and equipment, it has an increased life expectancy and probably will be used. Slides can be viewed easily with a handviewer and ambient light. Photographs can be held in the hand and several images, as with X rays, can be compared with each other. The audiotape cassette player is ubiquitous, easy-to-operate, and runs on batteries. If, however, the audiovisual material is immortalized in an integrated slide-tape show, a film, or videotape production, requiring equipment, special locations, and time to review, it will collect cobwebs. It is hoped that a convenient videotape format will be developed in the near future. If so, it will become the unifying audiovisual media, as it will be in color; it will produce still images that can be assessed separately, as well as moving images; and it will be small in size, playable on a small battery-powered or rechargeable unit; and will be relatively inexpensive.

Convenience to the Teacher

Audiotapes, photographs and slides, and videotapes are easy to make, revise, and duplicate. Complex media formats, such as film and integrated carrels, break down, require knowledge and patience to operate, require considerable maintenance, and are not conveniently available at most times.

Problem Unit Titles

This problem has been mentioned previously. Units need to be given titles, for cataloguing and retrieval. A system should be used that keeps the student unaware of the diagnosis or exact nature of the problem, or the value of the challenge offered to the student is diminished. Fictitious names, such as "Mary Jones," or serial codes in letters and numbers seem to be the only alternative to listing the problem units by diagnosis. If the problem's nature or diagnosis cannot be determined by its title, how does the teacher or student find an appropriate problem for study? Several possibilities exist.

Master Catalogue

This could be loose-leaf and describe each problem (in detail) by its code designation. A summary of the case, the data available on history, physical and laboratory tests, associated audiovisual material, and evaluation materials should be included. As time goes on, this catalogue could describe the accumulated results of student experience for the unit and suggestions for the teacher. Such a master catalogue allows the teacher to assemble the appropriate problems for both teaching and evaluation. It is of value to the teacher, but does not allow students to choose the appropriate problem for their own or their group's educational needs in a student-centered approach.

"Problem Finder"

This would have major headings organized around various basic science and clinical subject areas. Each would be subdivided under logical topic or content areas. In each of these, the problem that would stimulate both reasoning and study in these areas would be listed. This also could be designed as a chart, with clinical and basic science areas as one ordinate and the problems as another. This would allow student groups and students on self-study programs to choose appropriate problems.

Resource Librarian

Appoint a person in the curriculum or course who knows the available problems and can recommend appropriate problems to classes, student groups, individual students, or whatever, based on their stated educational objectives.

Problem-Based Learning Units versus Learning Resources

Such early problem-based learning resources as the "problem box" (Barrows & Mitchell, 1975) contained, in addition to the problem reference, lists suggesting a variety of resources, journal articles, monographs, test chapters, videotapes, slide-tape units, and films that the student might use as resources for further study. Occasionally, relevant reprints, diagrams, histological slides, and photographs also were included for the students' further study. The reference materials have been removed from our present use of the P4 and problem-box formats, however, for the following reasons.

1. Students felt that many of the references were too detailed and did not cover what they really wanted. They felt their time was wasted reading them.
2. The inclusion of superficial or overview references led to complaints that they were not of sufficient depth to be of value to the particular student.
3. After several years had passed, the faculty realized that many of the references were hopelessly out of date and many better ones had been published. Updating obviously had to be an annual chore with all problems.
4. It was realized that the inclusion of references took away the opportunity for the student to gain the appropriate skills of finding his own references, up-to-date and in sufficient scope, focus, and depth. This principal educational objective for medical students was being ignored!
5. The inclusion of references was a subtle intrusion of teacher-centered influence on the student.
6. The modest reference lists and collections in no way could compete with the treasures available in the medical library, where a vast array of references and "up-to-date" material was always available. Such references often were not thought of by faculty and were more likely to be relevant to particular students from any educational level or discipline.
7. As an alternative, appropriate faculty in the basic sciences and clinical specialties were identified in various parts of the curriculum as willing to help the student, if necessary, to find appropriate resources for his study.

Therefore, the terms *problem-based learning unit* and *learning resource* are used. The problem-based learning unit contains the patient problem (P4, problem box, PMP), associated audiovisual materials, and a variety of evaluation materials (issue lists, multiple-choice questions, reference patient write-ups, P4 flows, and so on). It requires updating only when new diagnostic tests or treatment approaches are appropriate for the problem. For example, some of the neuroscience problems existed before computerized transaxial tomography (CTT) was available; therefore, a CTT that would have occurred in the patient problem had to be added.

A learning resource is any source of stored information, usually subject-based, that the student can use for his problem-related learning, including books, journals, syllabi, monographs, audiovisual media units, models, cadavers, slides, and faculty. The use of resources can vary with the needs of the curriculum; the educational objectives; and the logistics involved in the numbers of students, their locations, and the facilities available. One or more of the following uses of learning resources may be appropriate.

1. No resources are made available, but the student has free run of the library and school.
2. A special room in the library or elsewhere is set aside for a collection of learning resources relevant for student study.
3. A transportable collection of resources is put near the area where students are working with the problem.

In addition, students often find it valuable to have a few appropriate texts nearby in their problem work so that they occasionally may look up information that is needed immediately, in order to move ahead with the problem, while noting down areas for later study.

Evaluation of Problem-Based Learning Units

It is essential that any problem-based learning unit be evaluated at many points in its development. When first designed, review by faculty, colleagues, and students can point out many problems and inconsistencies that have escaped the designer's notice. Students should be observed working with the unit, from the very beginning of their encounter to the end, to make certain they understand how it is to be used and to see if there are any assumptions they make about its use that may not have been identified.

There should be a form and a mechanism whereby students and faculty can report on their use of the unit, things they liked and didn't like, problems they had, and their suggestions.

Lastly, a more formal evaluation should be set up to see if the problem-based unit is able to meet the expected educational goals. The ways to do this depend on feasibility, time, cost and the evaluation tools available.

In conclusion, problem-based learning units feature a patient simulation in a manner that allows the student to develop all the important aspects of the clinical reasoning process. They are designed to facilitate self-directed study. They have tools included that allow for self-evaluation or faculty evaluation. They should be kept separate from learning resources that dispense subject-based information, and they should be evaluated.

CHAPTER 10

The Change to Problem-Based Learning

The most consistent and extensive application of problem-based/student-centered/self-directed learning in undergraduate education at the present time is in the school of medicine at McMaster University. Other medical schools at Michigan State University, Ohio State University, Southern Illinois University, and the University of Illinois also employ these techniques to some extent. The advantages of problem-based learning and self-directed study fit well into McMaster's objectives and their chosen learning format of small groups (usually five students) working with a member of the faculty ("tutor") in a facilitating role. There are no lecture series or courses in any of the standard disciplines of medical school and a pass–fail grading system is used. Year after year, this school holds workshops to improve the understanding and skills of the teaching faculty, particularly new faculty, and to improve and update the quality and number of formally designed problem-based learning units. It is in this environment that the authors have had considerable opportunity to gain experience in the development and application of problem-based learning and the approaches that help faculty and students gain the understanding and educational skills necessary for problem-based/student-centered/self-directed learning. The experience of this school, however, offers little help to an existing school or to new schools that may not have had the creative freedom that was possible at McMaster.

There is a variety of ways that individual problem-based learning units can be incorporated into existing curricula for schools that may wish to apply problem-based learning in some portions of their curriculum or as an alternative teaching approach in their schools. Problem-based learning units and simulated patients can be incorporated into a laboratory setting for groups of students, as part of a basic science course or as "laboratory work" in clinical medicine. Problem-based learning units can be incorporated directly into class work, with sufficient units provided for each student or small group of students. They also can be handed out to individual students or groups of students as outside assignments for larger discussion in the class setting. The problem-based units and simulated patients can be set up as correlative or integrated experiences for the students during clerkships, clinics, and in introductory clinical medicine courses, since they provide a natural transition to working with real patients. Problem-based learning units and simulated patients can be incorporated into an elective experience.

In the usual subject-based/teacher-centered courses, these units could be used easily as problems to amplify learning or to provide the students with experiences in the application of learned material to a patient problem. This would reinforce learning, increase student interest, and underline the relevance of the material to be learned. Most teachers should have little difficulty in seeing how problem-based units or patient simulations could be useful in their programs. This approach would not take full advantage of problem-based learning; however, if in these settings the problems were given to the students prior to the presentation or discussion of the basic or clinical information or concepts, their educational advantage would be realized better.

The problem addressed in this chapter is how a transition might be made to a truly problem-based/student-centered/self-directed study program as a teaching–learning format. A review of problem areas that must be considered will help faculty design strategies for change.

The Faculty

The majority of the teachers in the basic science and clinical faculty have been brought up through a traditional system of learning since kindergarten. It was the way most learned in their university, graduate school, or medical training. They know how to teach comfortably in a teacher-centered/subject-based system where they have responsibility for dispensing information, concepts, and skills in their discipline. Their positions of authority were hard won and they feel students must respect their expertise. As experts, they are keenly aware of how much students *must* know in the discipline they teach and how little time there is for students to cover it all. Lectures, demonstrations, and reading assignments seem to be the only way to get all that information covered.

Excellence in conventional teaching, accomplished through good lectures, brilliant seminars, or exciting patient rounds, is rewarded and builds reputations. There are few rewards given for efforts in innovative educational approaches or resource development. Tenure, promotion, and recognition resides with research, patient care, and administrative excellence. The ability to jump in and give a lecture or hold a seminar, lab, or clinic, and then leave, fits in well with these more demanding priorities. Lastly, the opportunity to develop new skills in teaching often is not attractive for someone who is already of academic rank. These factors must be recognized and appreciated. They require multiple approaches. One must create opportunities for the teacher to understand and become motivated about both the advantages of problem-based learning and the very natural aspect of the teaching skills required. Possible arenas include occasional educational rounds and departmental or school meetings. Another approach is to create a reward system for change and give recognition for innovative teaching activities, equal to research and patient care, and the time to carry them out. Approval and even pressure from chairmen and the deanery are important. This includes pressures to attend workshops on problem-based learning, teaching skills, and resource development. These approaches then can be reinforced by a successful pilot project in problem-based learning, which invariably develops student enthusiasm.

There is always a group in the faculty who learned by problems and by self-study, resisting tradition in their own education. They will gravitate to this approach and provide assistance. There are some in the faculty who are natural or intuitive facilitators of learning, who will help form a nucleus of support once they are oriented to problem-based learning. Find them!

The Students

There always is a number of students who will spontaneously opt for problem-based learning; however, there also is a group that will be very uncomfortable and threatened with this approach. Some in this latter group are just wary or insecure and may respond readily to an orientation concerning the educational advantages of problem-based learning and will work well with a teacher who has confidence and skills. Others resist due to ingrained, lifelong habits of wanting to read all about a subject before approaching any problem – a luxury they can't aford after graduation. Still others resist because they have very inadequate problem-solving capacities and could not adapt. The question can be raised as to whether these latter groups should go into medicine at all. They will have to be helped carefully, in order to survive in problem-based learning. Experience has shown repeatedly that students, in the majority, take to this approach like a duck to water and their enthusiasm tends to encourage other faculty and students to accept this approach. The elimination of grades by converting to a pass–fail system will help considerably, by eliminating competition for grades, and will tend to encourage students to help and teach each other, exchanging ideas and knowledge readily. It is essential, however, that pass–fail be based on rigorous and demanding criteria of performance and on careful evaluation. The other essential is the creation of a sense of openness about ignorance: students should feel free to say, "I don't know," so that they can learn. Traditional settings penalize students for admitting ignorance. This openness allows for effective self-directed learning and self-evaluation; plus a willingness to experiment and think openly. Obviously, the faculty also has to be able to say, "I don't know," and not feel threatened by such exposure.

Administrative Faculty

Encouragement and support from this sector are essential. Unfortunately, there have been many educational innovations that have been promoted for the sake of innovation, so they may be tired of hearing about any new educational approaches. Integrated teaching, ubiquitous and expensive (and usually unused) television facilities, free electives and visual formats of all kinds, and humanistic medicine are all examples. It is essential to provide for them an orientation to problem-based learning, its foundations and logic, and the studies and experiences that have occurred. They, as well as the teaching faculty, need to see a demonstration or to visit a school where problem-based learning is progressing. If there is one thing we have learned the hard way, year after year, it's that you will never achieve an understanding or enthusiasm for problem-based learning or problem simulation without a "hands on" demonstration in which faculty, students, and administrators are involved.

Time

Lectures, labs, seminars, clinics, and the like usually are carefully scheduled. For effective problem-based/self-directed learning, the student must be free to spend as little or as much time as he wishes working with problems, studying resources, talking with faculty, joining student discussions, and so forth. The time spent depends on the difficulties encountered and on the variety of learning activities undertaken in the self-study plan. To establish a problem-based learning curriculum there must be copious amounts of free time that is unscheduled for the student. This allows time to be budgeted by each individual student or student group to meet their particular study plans, priorities, and approaches. To be individualized and student-centered, it has to be free and unstructured, so the individual student can structure it appropriately. This underlines the responsibility given to the student for his education.

Not only should the time be free, it also should avoid any competition with a structured, teacher-centered, traditionally based course. As an example, a relatively new school mounted a problem-based individualized study course in neuroscience that provided the student with unstructured time, for study and work with problems, every morning of the week for a number of weeks. In the afternoon, the students took lectures and labs in biochemistry, with midterms, finals, required lab reports, and unscheduled exams. The result was that the immediate short-term concerns and anxieties about the lab reports, exams, and grades caused the free and unstructured time to be used up studying biochemistry. This deprived students of the chance to realize the advantages of having their own time to work toward more valuable, long-term goals. These parallel courses probably would be handled well by students well-versed and confident in problem-based, self-directed study; however, this is no way to get such a program off of the ground. The faculty and students need to be able to relax and adjust to the change in responsibility and approach. When this course changed to a day-long block of time, for fewer weeks, the students spent their time appropriately.

Learning Resources

With scheduled classes in specific subjects, the learning resources that are needed can be specified. The assigned texts, monographs, slides, models, specimens, and demonstrations can be obtained. The faculty all have scheduled times to present a specific subject or topic to the students. In short, the needed learning resources for the entire class can be specified ahead of time and any demands outside of such focused requirements are slight. In self-directed/problem-based learning, students, either in groups or alone, go off in their different ways to study the resources of all varieties that they feel are appropriate to meet the school's and their own educational objectives. This is not necessarily chaos, since the problems encountered by the students may be in a particular subject area, such as cardiology, primary care, anatomy, or pathology, and the range of self-directed study has its boundaries. Even if the problems are taken on as an introduction to medicine, each problem emphasizes certain disciplines and areas. This requires the faculty to amass a wide range of appropriate resources that are available at most times for the students to use. This larger range of resources needed by students on self-study programs has to be anticipated, since as it can affect the library, slide stores, laboratory facilities, and clinical resources.

During the adoption of a program in problem-based learning, the school is in a double-demand system, in which syllabi, books, specimens, and equipment are utilized in the usual peak-and-through patterns, and in which almost anything may be wanted at any time.

All of this can be handled effectively if anticipated. Problems can be taken in a different order by different students or groups, so that they do not all demand the same learning resources related to one problem at the same time. Secondly, the availability of some resources can be scheduled so that they are available certain hours of certain days; the self-study students can schedule themselves accordingly. A separate library can be stocked with a range of relevant resources set aside for these students, with a seven-day-a-week availability.

Faculty Resources

The input of time necessary to meet with students as a facilitator of problem-based learning is not as great as usually assumed. The experience at McMaster would suggest that no more than six hours or so a week may be necessary. This must be scheduled by the individual faculty–student group. The time advantage in self-directed study is that the student takes on many of the responsibilities of the teacher. The teacher facilitates, monitors, stimulates, and periodically evaluates. The resource faculty, or the experts on the faculty in the basic sciences and clinical sciences whom the student may want to consult as a resource for self-study information in their field, can be made available on a scheduled basis. For example, a hematologist might be available for seminars or talks with students during a period students are working with hematological problems, say, on Mondays and Wednesdays from 10–12 A.M. At that time, he could schedule himself to be in one place, doing interruptable work, so that if students do not show up he hasn't wasted time. Again, there are many ways this can be handled. The important thing is the awareness of the problem.

Despite this, the teaching faculty for problem-based learning will have to be free to devote energies to starting such a program. No one on the faculty will be able to give scheduled lectures or supervise a lab and at the same time be available to develop problem-based, self-study groups. Some faculty will have to be given the time and incentives to collect, assemble, or design and construct problem-based learning units, learning resources, and evaluation tools. There has to be the commitment of time and effort from other faculty in related departments, basic or clinical, to serve as advisors or consultants in the preparation of these resources and to help in designing objectives and evaluation criteria.

The Appropriate Model

A pilot for problem-based learning might occur within a departmental group that has a block of time in the curriculum long enough (six to eight weeks) to attempt problem-based learning. This could be in a basic science course, an integrated course (neuroscience), a departmental course (pathology or pediatrics), or in a special interdepartmental course (introduction to clinical medicine). An undesirable effect of a single block of problem-based learning is that as soon as the students develop the ability to carry out problem-based/self-directed learning and accept responsibility for their own education, the block is finished and they plunge back into their regular curriculum. The positive effects of the experience soon may be lost unless the students carry on with problem-based learning on their own. The desirable effect is that the students will, if it is done well, become enthusiastic about the experience and other faculty may be encouraged to try similar approaches. This allows all faculty and students to see such a teaching–learning approach in action.

Another model would be to set up a parallel or alternative curriculum that was problem-based and self-directed. This is far more ambitious and complex. It has the advantage of continuity toward accomplishing in the graduating student the objectives set for problem-based learning (see Chapter 1). The curriculum at McMaster University and the proposed curriculum in primary care at the University of New Mexico can be reviewed as models for such an undertaking. The latter proposed many of the evaluation techniques described in Chapter 7, and the regular medical school will serve as the control group.

The easiest pilot would be an elective experience in problem-based/self-directed learning. This would have less impact for change, since the faculty might not see how it could be incorporated into the regular curriculum and the motivation or progress of the students would be hard to measure in comparison to anything else because they selected themselves by their interest in such an elective.

The impetus to problem-based learning can start at either an administrative or a "grass roots" level, gaining the enthusiasm and support of students and faculty for a pilot program. In some schools, groups of students and some faculty start problem-based/self-directed study groups during spare hours, to expand their understanding and ability to apply information from the particular section of the curriculum they are in. This leads, in turn, to visits to schools using this method and, finally, to a pilot program in the curriculum. Students can carry the impetus for change a long way, but, without faculty help, it is pointless; the students move on every year and their experiences go with them. The willingness of deans or departmental chairmen to attempt problem-based learning works only as long as the cooperation and skills of the faculty also are developed. A good method for achieving the latter is to have recurrent faculty and student workshops on a variety of areas in problem-based learning. The subjects of these workshops could include facilitating group learning, teaching and evaluating clinical reasoning with patient simulations, problem-based learning unit designs and use, training and use of simulated patients, and learning resource design. Participation by students and the direct experience by the faculty in the true "workshop" sense is important.

In summary, the following points need to be met in designing a unit of instruction that features problem-based learning and self-directed study.

1. Sufficient instructional time
2. Absence of a competing instructional program that makes unfair demands on the students
3. Preparation of adequate learning resources for self-directed study
4. Adequate resource faculty
5. Well-defined goals and evaluation techniques that are visible to both faculty and students
6. Adequate orientation of faculty and students
7. Recurrent faculty workshops (with student participation).

CHAPTER **11**

A Summary

Difficulties in the Application of Problem-Based Learning

The majority of the difficulties that occur in the application of problem-based learning are the result of poor understanding, by students or teachers, of the process as a whole.

Many times, students will not take on the problem as an unknown because they feel they must have some background knowledge in the area in order to work with the problem. Instead, they will review texts in the area of the problem before it is encountered. They run the risk of wasting considerable time in study that will be of no value with the specific problem and of not studying what will turn out to be important. One of the major advantages of problem-based learning is lost in this inefficient approach. The student can determine what he already knows and what he really needs to learn only if the problem is taken on first. In doing this, he develops as far as possible his skills in reasoning with an unfamiliar problem. The student's self-study is focused better and is more likely to meet his personal needs, and the information sought is seen as relevant and probably more memorable if the student takes on the problem first.

Another problem occurs when the students read through or review a problem to determine the necessary learning issues, without actually trying to determine how they would evaluate and manage the problem themselves. Although this is almost impossible to do with a simulated patient, real patient, or P4, it is easy to do with a sequential management problem, patient management problem, or case history. Again, the students do not take on the challenge of reasoning through the problem, of finding out what they really need to know in order to understand or to manage such a problem, and of discovering how adequate their skills are in evaluating the problem. The problem is used merely as a sign to indicate, by the nature of its content, what subject areas might be reviewed. This certainly is not problem-based learning, and the student is deprived of its impact.

As suggested by the previous paragraph, poorly designed problems for problem-based learning can defeat the whole approach, unless the teacher adapts them before student contact. There is no point in belaboring this; several chapters have been devoted to the proper design and choice of problem formats.

Another significant problem occurs when the students do not apply what they have learned back to the problem, to see if, as a consequence, the problem can be understood and/or managed better. This is essential, as it reinforces what has been learned through application and ensures recall of that knowledge when confronted by a similar problem. The students also must go the last mile and review what they learned and how it integrates with what they already know, before taking on the next problem.

Other areas of difficulty usually relate to insecurity on the part of the teacher, who still feels that problem-based learning is inefficient and that, for some reason, his students should receive a systematized body of knowledge about his discipline. Again, "efficiency" in this context refers to the acquisition of facts; the teacher fails to see that the time involved in working with the problem, in self-directed study, and in the application of information back to the problem allows the student to acquire much more than facts. If the teacher would think about his own behavior, he might drop the concern about "systematized knowledge." If he had to give a lecture tomorrow on a topic in his field, he would have to review some papers or texts tonight to "organize" his thoughts; yet he is perfectly capable today of handling any patient problem in that topic area. If the knowledge he needs is not systematized, why should an external system be forced on the student? In addition, every professor around the world would organize or systematize the same topic in a different way, each including or excluding different facts, developing slightly different concepts, and organizing the subject matter differently. The student should be able to organize information any way he wishes, to suit his style and needs and to facilitate his analysis and understanding.

A Summary of the Process of Problem-Based Learning

1. The problem is encountered first in the learning sequence, before any preparation or study has occurred.
2. The problem situation is presented to the student in the same way it would present in reality.
3. The student works with the problem in a manner that permits his ability to reason and apply knowledge to be challenged and evaluated, appropriate to his level of learning.
4. Needed areas of learning are identified in the process of work with the problem and used as a guide to individualized study.

5. The skills and knowledge acquired by this study are applied back to the problem, to evaluate the effectiveness of learning and to reinforce learning.
6. The learning that has occurred in work with the problem and in individualized study is summarized and integrated into the student's existing knowledge and skills.

A Summary of the Process of Clinical Reasoning

The clinician:

1. Perceives initial cues from the patient and environment
2. Rapidly generates multiple hypotheses
3. Applies an inquiry strategy (questions, examinations, tests) to refine, rank, verify, and eliminate hypotheses
4. Abstracts an enlarging problem formulation from the significant hypothesis-related data obtained from ongoing inquiry
5. Closes the encounter when he has made diagnostic and therapeutic decisions.

This is the process that the student should apply at point 3 in the problem-based learning process.

A Summary of the Process of Self-Directed Study

1. During the problem encounter, all questions, insecurities, or holes in knowledge should be noted down as learning issues.
2. Whenever work with the problem has to stop due to lack of knowledge or understanding, the learning issues should be reviewed and a study plan devised, relative to the goals of the curriculum.
3. The study plan should be sensitive to the specific learning needs and background of the learner.
4. Learning resources can be *books, monographs, journals,* cadavers, specimens, models, *faculty experts,* field trips, and audiovisual units, as appropriate (those emphasized are available to physicians generally).
5. At an agreed time, the learning acquired will be brought back to the problem.

A Summary of the Educational Advantages of Problem-Based Learning

Problem-based/student-centered learning, used as defined, offers educational advantages in the light of the objectives that concern the development of clinical reasoning, patient evaluation and care, and self-education.

1. Clinical reasoning (problem-solving) skills can be learned and evaluated.
2. Through the context of working with the problem, a student can discover personal educational needs relevant to his career in medicine.
3. Information is learned in the context of trying to understand a patient problem, facilitating recall and transfer of that information in work with future related problems.
4. Information is reinforced through reuse.
5. Information from many disciplines is integrated in the mind of the learner.
6. Learning is seen by the student as being relevant.
7. Students are actively involved and motivated.
8. Self-evaluation and self-learning skills are learned and evaluated.
9. Students can be treated as adults responsible for their own learning.

The primary objective of problem-based learning is to give the student skills and information that he will transfer to his work with real patients, both as he is learning and for the rest of his professional life. It is hoped that he not only will develop and apply efficient and effective reasoning skills with his patients, but will use each patient experience as an evaluation of what he needs to learn and will engage in continual self-study to keep his knowledge and skills contemporary and appropriate to his tasks.

This learning approach can be modified for educational tasks in continuing medical education, learning in other health professions, and in team learning. It is particularly effective for the latter because the patient is the focus of any health team and a simulated patient problem allows for members of a health-care team to learn to coordinate their individualized approaches around the patient problem. It also permits them to carry out study, as appropriate, in their own disciplines and bring what they have learned back to the problem, for the rest to consider.

References

Abrahamson, S., Presentation on SIM 1 at the Symposium and Exhibition on New Developments in Medical Technology at the University of Limburg, Maastricht, The Netherlands. June 1978.

Anderson, B. F., *Cognitive Psychology*. Academic Press, New York, 1975.

Arnheim, R., *Visual Thinking*. University of California Press, Berkeley, 1969.   *p 41*

Barro, A. R., Survey and Evaluation of Approaches to Physician Performance Measurement. *Journal of Medical Education* 48(11):1047–1087, November 1973.

Barrows, H. S., *Simulated Patients*. Charles C Thomas, Springfield, Ill., 1971.

Barrows, H. S., and Abrahamson, S., The Programmed Patient: A Technique for Appraising Student Performance in Clinical Neurology. *Journal of Medical Education* 39(8):802–805, August 1964.

Barrows, H. S., and Bennett, K., Experimental Studies on the Diagnostic (Problem Solving) Skill of the Neurologist, Their Implications for Neurological Training. *Archives of Neurology* 26(3):273–277, March 1972.   *p 20*

Barrows, H. S., and Mitchell, D. L. M., An Innovative Course in Undergraduate Neuroscience Experiment in Problem Based Learning with "Problem Boxes." *British Journal of Medical Education* 9(4):223–230, December 1975.

Barrows, H. S., and Tamblyn, R. M., An Evaluation of Problem Based Learning in Small Groups Utilizing a Simulated Patient. *Journal of Medical Education* 51(1):52–54, January 1976. (a)

Barrows, H. S., and Tamblyn, R. M., Self-Assessment Units. *Journal of Medical Education* 51(4):334–336, April 1976. (b)

Barrows, H. S., and Tamblyn, R. M., The Portable Patient Problem Pack (P4): A Problem Based Learning Unit. *Journal of Medical Education* 52(12): 1002–1004, December 1977.

195

p²¹ Barrows, H. S., Feightner, J. W., Neufeld, V. R., and Norman, G. R., Analysis of the clinical Methods of Medical Students and Physicians. Supported by Ontario Department of Health, Grants ODH-PR-273 and ODH-DM-226. McMaster University, Hamilton, Ontario, Canada, 1978.

p²⁰ Barrows, H. S., Tamblyn, R. M., Sinclair, J. C., Watts, J. L., Mohide, P. T., Kaufman, K. S., Leitch, R. E., Conlin, M. S., Milner, R. S., Elliot, M. J., and Anderson, G. D., A Problem Based, Self Directed Educational Program in Neonatal Respiratory Disease for Community Hospital Personnel. Proceedings of the 17th Annual Conference on Research in Medical Education, New Orleans, pp. 111-116, 1978.

Bartlett, F. C., *Thinking*. Basic Books, New York, 1958.

Bashook, P. G., A Conceptual Framework for Measuring Clinical Problem Solving. *Journal of Medical Education* 51(2):110-114, February 1976.

Berner, E. S., Hamilton, L. S., and Best, W. R., A New Approach to Evaluating Problem Solving in Medical Students. *Journal of Medical Education* 49(7):666-672, July 1974.

p²¹ Burri, A., McCaughan, K., and Barrows, H. S., The Feasibility of Using the Simulated Patient as a Means to Evaluate Clinical Competence of Physicians in a Community (A Pilot Project). Proceedings of the Fifteenth Annual Conference on Research in Medical Education, San Francisco, pp. 295-299, Nov. 13-14, 1976.

p²¹ Campbell, E. J. M., Clinical Science. *Clinical Science and Molecular Medicine* 51(12):1-7, December 1976.

p²¹ Chamberlain, T. C., The Method of Multiple Working Hypotheses. (Reprinted from Science 15:92, 1890). *Science* 148(5):754-759, May 1965.

Denson, J. S., and Abrahamson, S., Computer Controlled Patient Simulation. *Journal of the American Medical Association* 208(4):504-508, April 1969.

de Bono, E., *The Five-Day Course in Thinking*. Penguin Books, Baltimore, 1969.

de Dombal, F. T., Smith, R. B., Modgill, V. K., and Leaper, D. J., Simulation of the Diagnostic Process: A Further Comparison. *British Journal of Medical Education* 6(3):238-245, September 1972.

Dickinson, C. J., Goldsmith, C. H., and Sackett, D. L., MacMan: A Digital Computer Model for Teaching Some Basic Principles of Hemodynamics. *Journal of Clinical Computing* 2(1):42-50, January 1973.

Echt, R., and Chan, S., A New Problem-Oriented and Student-Centered Curriculum at Michigan State University. *Journal of Medical Education* 52(8):681-683, August 1977.

p²¹ Elstein, A. S., Shulman, L. S., and Sprafka, S. S., *An Analysis of Clinical Reasoning*. Harvard University Press, Cambridge, MA., 1978.

p²¹ Elstein, A. S., Kagan, N., Shulman, L. S., Jason, H. and Loupe, M. J., Methods and Theory in the Study of Medical Inquiry. *Journal of Medical Education* 47(2):85-92, February 1972.

Feightner, J. W., Barrows, H. S., Neufeld, V. R., and Norman, G. R., Solving Problems: How Does the Family Physician Do It? *Canadian Family Physician* 23(457):67-71, April 1977.

Feightner, J. W., and Norman, G. R., Concurrent Validity of Patient Management Problems by Comparison with the Clinical Encounter. Proceedings of the 15th Conference on Research in Medical Education, San Francisco, pp. 149-154, Nov. 13-14, 1976.

Friedman, R. B., A Computer Programme for Simulating the Patient-Physician Encounter? *Journal of Medical Education* 48(1):92-97, January 1973.

Friedman, R. B., Newsom, R. S., Entine, S. M., Summing, C., and Schultz, J. V., A Simulated Patient-Physician Encounter Using a Talking Computer. *Journal of the American Medical Association* 238(10):1927-1929, October 1977.

Goran, M. J., Williamson, J. W., and Gonnella, J. S., The Validity of Patient Management Problems. *Journal of Medical Education* 48(2):171-177, February 1973.

Gordon, M. S., Cardiology Patient Simulator. *American Journal of Cardiology* 34(9):350, September 1974.

Harden, R. McG., Stevenson, M., Downie, W. W., and Wilson, G. M., Assessment of Clinical Competence Using Objective Structured Examination. *British Medical Journal* 1(2):447-451, February 1975.

Harless, W. G., Drennon, G. G., Marxer, J. J., Root, J. A., and Miller, G. E., CASE: A Computer Aided Simulation of the Clinical Encounter. *Journal of Medical Education* 46(5):443-448, May 1971.

Helfer, R. E., and Slater, C. H., Measuring the Process of Solving Clinical Diagnostic Problems. *British Journal of Medical Education* 5(1):48-52, March 1971.

Hilgard, E. R., Irvine, R. P., and Whipple, J. E., Rote Memorization, Understanding, and Transfer: An Extension of Katona's Card Trick Experiments. *Journal of Experimental Psychology* 46(4):288-292, April 1953.

Hodgkin, K., and Knox, J. D. E., *Problem Centered Learning.* Churchill Livingstone, Edinburgh, London, and New York, 1975.

Hubbard, J. P., Levit, E. J., Schumacher, C. F., and Schnabel, T. G., An Objective Evaluation of Clinical Competence. *New England Journal of Medicine* 272(25):1321-1328, June 1965.

Jason, H., Kagan, N., Werner, A., Elstein, A., and Thomas, J. B., New Approaches to Teaching Basic Interview Skills to Medical Students. *American Journal of Psychiatry* 127(10):1404-1407, April 1971.

Johnson, M. L. A., *The Anatomy of Judgement*. Penguin Books, London, 1943.

P28

Kassirer, J. P., Gorry, G. A., Clinical Problem Solving: A Behavioral Analysis. *Anals of Internal Medicine* 89(8):245-255, August 1978.

Katona, G., *Organizing and Memorizing*. Columbia University Press, New York, 1940.

Keller, F. S., Good-Bye Teacher . . . . *Journal of Applied Behaviour Analysis* 1:79-89, Spring 1968.

p21

Kleinmuntz, B., *The Processing of Clinical Information by Man and Machine.* Chapter VI, The Formal Representation of Human Judgment. Carnegie-Mellon University, 1968.

Knowles, M., *Self Directed Learning: A Guide for Learners and Teachers.* Association Press, New York, 1975.

Leaper, D. J., Gill, P. W., Staniland, J. R., Harrocks, J. C., and de Dombal, F. T., Clinical Diagnostic Process: An Analysis. *British Medical Journal* 3(9):569-574, September 1973.

Levine, H. G., and Forman, P. M., A Study of Retention of Knowledge of Neurosciences Information. *Journal of Medical Education* 48(9):867-869, September 1973.

p41

Luria, A. R., *The Working Brain: An Introduction to Neuropsychiatry.* Penguin Books, New York, 1973.

Maatch, J. L., *An Introduction to Patient Games: Some Fundamentals of Clinical Introduction.* Biomedical Communications Center, Michigan State University, 1974.

Mager, R. F., *Measuring Instructional Intent or Got a Match?* Fearon Publishers, Belmont, CA., 1973.

p20

McGuire, C. H., Research on Identification of Student Needs. Proceedings of the Fourth Panamerican Conference on Medical Education, Toronto, Ontario, Canada, pp. 154-160, August 28-30, 1972.

McGuire, C. H., and Babbott, D., Simulation Technique in the Measurement of Problem Solving Skills. *Journal of Educational Measurement* 4(1): Spring 1967.

McWhinney, I. R., Problem Solving and Decision Making in Primary Medical Practice. *Proceedings of the Royal Society of Medicine* 65:34-38, 1972.

p26

Mechanic, D., and Parson, W., Editorial: Shortcuts Are Not Necessarily Bad. *Journal of Medical Education* 50(6):638-639, June 1975.

P21

Medawar, P. B., *Introduction and Intuition in Scientific Thought.* Methuen, London, 1969.

P6

Miller, G. E., Continuing Medical Education for What? *MCV Quarterly* 3(3):152-156, 1967. (a)

Miller, G. E., Continuous Assessment. *Medical Education* 10:81-86, 1976.

Miller, G. E., The Contributions of Research in the Learning Process. *Medical Education* 12(5):28, May 1978.

Miller, G. E., Educational Science and Education for Medicine. *British Journal of Medical Education* 1(3):156-159, June 1967. (b)

Miller, G. E., An Inquiry into Medical Teaching. *Journal of Medical Education* 37(3):185-191, March 1962.

Miller, G. A., The Magical Number Seven, Plus or Minus Two: Some Limits on Our Capacity for Processing Information. *Psychology Review* 63:81-97, 1956.

Murray, T. J., Relevance in Undergraduate Neurological Teaching. *Canadian Journal of Neurological Sciences* 4(2):131-137, May 1977.

Neufeld, V. R., and Barrows, H. S., The "McMaster Philosophy": An Approach to Medical Education. *Journal of Medical Education* 49(11): 1040-1050, November 1974.

Newble, D., *The Evaluation of Clinical Competence.* The University of Adelaide, Department of Medicine, 1975.

Obenshain, S., Kaufman, A., Voorhees, J. D., and Burrola, N., *The Curriculum for Primary Care Program.* The University of New Mexico, School of Medicine, 1978.

Pauker, S. G., Gorry, G. A., Kassirer, J. P., and Schwartz, W. B., Towards the Simulation of Clinical Cognition: Taking a Present Illness by Computer. *American Journal of Medicine* 60(2):981-996, June 1976.

Platt, J. R., Strong Inference. *Science* 146(10):347-353, October 1964.

Rimoldi, H. J. A., Problem Solving. Proceedings of the Fourth Panamerican Conference on Medical Education, Toronto, Ontario, Canada, pp. 117-129, August 1972.

Rimoldi, H. J. A., The Test of Diagnostic Skills. *Journal of Medical Education* 36:73-79, January 1973.

Sandok, B. A., Another New Neuroscience Program. Paper included in the course booklet for Neurological Education at the American Academy of Neurology meeting, pp. 127-135, April 25-30, 1977.

Schmidt, W. H. O., Processes of Learning in Relation to Different Kinds of Materials to Be Learnt. In *Medical Education in South Africa,* J. V. O. Reid and A. J. Wilmot, eds., Natal University Press, Pietermaritzburg, South Africa, 1965, pp. 228-232. (Note: This is the proceedings of the Conference on Medical Education held at the University of Natal, Durban, South Africa, July 1964. It contains individual papers by title, with no chapters, and is published in hard bound form.)

Sinclair, J. C., Experimental Design Deck for Clinical Research: A New Learning Resource in Aid of Scientific Thinking. *Pediatrics* 62(5):981-996, May 1978.

Spitzer, W., Sackett, D. L., and Sibley, J. C., The Burlington Randomized

Trial of the Nurse Practitioner. *New England Journal of Medicine* 290(1):251–256, January 1974.

Tamblyn, R. M., and Barrows, H., Evaluation Trial of the P4 System (Portable Patient Problem Pack), Problem Based Learning Systems Monograph #4. Supported by Contract NO1–LM–6–4721, National Library of Medicine, Bethesda, Maryland, 1978, (To be published in *Medical Education*).

Weed, L. L., *Medical Records, Medical Education and Patient Care.* Case Western Reserve University Press, 1969.

West, K. M., The Case against Teaching. *Journal of Medical Education* 41(8): 766–771, August 1966.

Williamson, J. W., Assessing Clinical Judgement. *Journal of Medical Education* 40(2):180–187, February 1965.

Wingard, J. R., and Williamson, J. W., Grades as Predictors of Physician's Career Performance: An Evaluative Literature Review. *Journal of Medical Education* 48(4):311–332, April 1973.

Index